BONES OF IRON

COLLECTED ARTICLES ON THE LIFE OF THE STRENGTH ATHLETE

MATT FOREMAN

Printed in the United States of America
10 9 8 7 6 5 4 3 2 1

ISBN-13: 978-0-9800111-2-8
ISBN-10: 0-9800111-2-4

Articles first published in the
Performance Menu: Journal of Health & Athletic Excellence

Catalyst Athletics, Inc.
www.cathletics.com

BONES OF IRON

COLLECTED ARTICLES ON THE LIFE OF THE STRENGTH ATHLETE

MATT FOREMAN

To my parents, for everything

CONTENTS

INTRODUCTION

When you read the articles in this book, you're going to find a lot of quotes and references from famous films and books. I'm a movie buff and a big reader, so I connect a lot of scenes and one-liners to the subjects I write about. I guess we'll start this introduction with something a lot of you will probably recognize. In the 80s movie *Wall Street*, yuppie wanna-be Bud Fox is preparing for his first big meeting with financial tyrannosaurus Gordon Gekko. Fox knows that Gekko could make him a rich man by giving him a job, and right before he walks into Gekko's office for the first time, he looks in a mirror and says, "Life all comes down to a few moments. This is one of them."

Bud understood that there are a handful of decisions we all make in our lives that ultimately determine everything about our time on this earth. The choices we make when we select a career, get married, have/don't have children, etc. are the moments Bud was talking about. When we grow old, we look back on our lives and realize the impact that followed these decisions. And I can absolutely, positively tell you that one of those crucial moments in my life happened in May 1988 when I decided to compete in my first powerlifting meet

I was a little loser at that point in my life. I was fifteen, straight-D student, borderline juvenile delinquent, the whole package. I joined the freshman football team because I thought it would be a good way to get chicks. Our coaches made us lift weights, I was stronger than most of the guys on the team right away, and after a year I decided that it would be pretty cool to compete in a lifting meet. So without any coaching, direction, or comprehension of what I was doing, I entered the 1988 Arizona State High School Powerlifting Championships and broke the state record in the deadlift my first time out. It's funny to think back about that day because I actually knew right then that my whole life had changed. Even though I was young and basically an idiot, I understood that I had found something. I had a fever, and the only prescription was bigger lifts.

I competed as a powerlifter for two more years and then converted to Olympic Weightlifting. It took me a lot longer to become successful in this new sport, but I eventually got the hang of it and started working my way up the mountain.

Now, here we are over two decades later, and being a competitive strength athlete and multi-sport coach have become the foundations of my life. I've had a terrific career with a lot of peaks and valleys, and I've met some of the best people of my life in the iron game. Back in 2008, I was lucky enough to meet Greg Everett and Aimee Anaya. All three of us were competing at the California State Games, and we hit it off right away. It wasn't long after this meet that Greg asked me to write an article for an online magazine he published called The Performance Menu. I accepted his offer, he liked what I wrote, and we decided to keep going with it on a monthly basis.

Here we are, almost three years later, and writing articles for Greg and Aimee's magazine has been a fascinating side project for me. I've learned so many lessons throughout my career in strength athletics, and The Performance Menu has given me an opportunity to put these lessons out to the public in the hope that others will be able to enrich their lifting lives through reading them. Many of these articles have been about the nuts-and-bolts training of a weightlifter, general strength athlete, CrossFitter, etc. People read the magazine because they want to learn better ways to get strong, so that has been the main focus. However, I've also written several articles about the experiences I've had and the philosophies I've developed. They're in here too. Additionally, I've included some short vignette material that hasn't been read by anybody yet. These are quick little scenes that describe a special moment, person, or some kind of insight that left a mark on me. Some are funny and some are serious. They're peppered around the book; you'll know them when you see them.

The greatest reward I could imagine would be to know that other lifters and coaches have learned something valuable in this book and then paid it forward by using that learning to make other people better. I hope you enjoy reading this as much as I've enjoyed writing it. And I especially hope you enjoy living the life of iron as much as I've enjoyed mine.

—*Matt Foreman*

SECTION ONE: TRAINING

This first section will take up the majority of the book, and the focus is on a wide range of strength training issues. Most of what I've written has leaned towards the specific training of an Olympic weightlifter. However, I've always been conscious that many of the people who read Performance Menu are "strength generalists." I just started hearing this term a few years ago and it makes a lot of sense to describe a person who incorporates the Olympic lifts into a diverse program that is designed to produce the highest overall strength capacity. Whether you're a competitive lifter or just somebody who uses the Olympic lifts as a component of your training, you'll find something in this section that will make you better. Technique, programming, injury management, exercise selection… it's all in here.

THESE GO UP TO ELEVEN: PLANNING APPROPRIATE TRAINING VOLUME FOR WEIGHTLIFTERS

First of all, we need to agree that if you haven't seen the movie *This is Spinal Tap*, you're just letting the best things in life slip through your fingers.

In the heavy metal spoof, Spinal Tap guitarist Nigel Tufnel is showing an interviewer the amplifier he uses when he plays his guitar. The most important detail of the amp, as Nigel points out, is that the volume dials all go up to a maximum setting of "11" instead of just the normal 10. Nigel explains that when the band is really rocking hard and they need a massive burst of power, they crank the dial up to 11 for that "extra push over the cliff." What Nigel and the band were looking for was VOLUME! They needed to smash through the barrier of a normal amp's volume and really go for heavy metal madness, so their amps needed special dials. If none of this sounds funny or you don't get the point, my apologies.

However, Nigel and the other members of Spinal Tap were obsessed with volume, and this is where the common ground with weightlifting can be found. Over the years, I've come to believe that planning the appropriate amount of training volume for weightlifters and other athletes is probably one of the most difficult and extremely important factors in any sport. Coaches and athletes wrestle throughout the year with the question "How much is too much?" When we talk about volume, obviously, we're talking about the amount of exercises, sets, and reps that are performed by the athletes during their workouts and how many workouts take place in a week, month, etc. Everyone has learned that athletes have to work hard and push themselves if they want to be successful, but it is also equally clear to anyone with experience that pushing too hard will lead to burnout and injury. If athletes don't have enough volume in their training programs, they will never make the progress they're capable of because they aren't working hard enough. If athletes have too much volume in their training programs, they will battle injuries constantly because their bodies cannot endure all the punishment.

Therefore, there is a fine line of perfect volume that has to be discovered when a coach/athlete plans out a workout regimen. And that "fine line" is a slippery little sucker because each athlete has different physical qualities and, therefore, different volume capabilities. Human beings vary greatly in areas like testosterone production, bone density, connective tissue durability, emotional toughness, and muscle recovery speed. To put it more simply, the optimal level of volume for each athlete will be individualized, and the coach who writes the training programs for the athletes has to make adjustments in order to avoid injuries.

A good way to analyze this area is to look at two different extremes. One of those extremes will be the training volume of the most powerful weightlifting country in the world right now... China. The other extreme will be the training volume of an aging American lifter who is finding ways to extend his career with little more than muscle memory and a handsome face.

The Red Goliath of the East

Chinese lifters won eight gold medals at the 2008 Beijing Olympics. Chinese lifters demolish world records. China has become a phenomenal weightlifting powerhouse, and you're not going to read a detailed analysis of their training system in this article because there is an element of secrecy involved with their success. Chinese communist culture, as with all communist systems, never reveals all the hidden elements of their country to the world. The Chinese don't operate under a complete black cloak of mystery, but they also make sure the whole world isn't privy to the nuts and bolts of their operation. Knowing this, what can we say for certain about their program?

A former Chinese coach once told me that there are over a million registered weightlifters in China. With that kind of talent pool, along with their fantastically organized sports academy system (funded by the government) that channels young athletes into full-time training from an early age, they are playing with a different set of rules. So, if this article is focused on training volume, how much volume do their athletes use in their training?

I don't know for sure, but there is something I know for sure that can give us some solid ideas. At the Beijing Olympics, the women's 75 kilo class was won by China's Cao Lei. Cao snatched 128 kilos and clean and jerked 154 kilos, winning the class with a 282 kilo total (16 kilos more than the silver medalist). First of all, you need to get your mind around the idea that a 165 pound woman snatched 282 pounds and clean & jerked 339. After you've recovered, remember that Cao's performance was mediocre because the Chinese woman who won the 69 kilo class (one weight class lighter than Cao) totaled 286 kilos.

Please don't quit, it's going to be okay...

A reporter for World Weightlifting magazine took notes as Cao warmed up for her competition attempts at the Olympics. Here is her warm-up progression for the snatch:

Snatch	Weight (in kilos)
1st	15
2nd	15
3rd	35x2
4th	35x2
5th	45x2
6th	45x2
7th	65x1
8th	75x2
9th	75x2
10th	85x2
12th	95x2
13th	95x2
14th	100x2
15th	105x2
16th	110x2
17th	110x2
18th	115x1
19th	115x1
20th	120x1
21st	120x1
22nd	120x1
1st Attempt	120
2nd Attempt	125
3rd Attempt	128

This information was documented by an eyewitness, and you read it correctly. Cao took 22 warm-up sets in the snatch, and she actually snatched her competition opener of 120 kilos three times in the warm-up room before taking the platform and going three-for-three with 120, 125, 128. To conserve space in this article, I won't go through her warm-up progression for the clean and jerk, but she took eighteen warm-up sets for that lift. She clean & jerked 145 two times in the warm-up room before her competition opener of 147 kilos. She made 147, 154, and missed 159 on her third attempt.

Side note: Cao's failure at 159 was the only failed attempt by any Chinese woman at the Olympics. All of their other women made six flawless attempts. Interestingly, Cao stated that she had missed 159 due to a "mental lapse." She attributed the mental lapse to the death of her mother shortly before the Olympics. Chinese lifters live full-time in training camps and they are rarely allowed to see their families, so the Chinese government withheld the news of her mother's death because they did not want to distract her training. Right before the games, her coach decided to tell Cao of her mother's demise. Another Chinese Olympic

Champion, Liu Chunhong of the 69 kilos class, stated in a post-meet interview that she had only been allowed to see her family for a week after the 2004 Athens Olympics before she went back to training camp. She was grateful for her 2008 gold medal because she was going to be allowed to see her family again after the Games. Think about these little details when you think about how hard the Chinese train.

Back to Cao Lei: Taking 22 warm-up attempts in the snatch, including three warm-up attempts at her competition opener, is beyond the realm of normal weightlifting comprehension. This is the most jaw-dropping example of work capacity that I have ever heard of because, as we know, an athlete's warm-up progression at a major competition will always be designed to conserve some energy and keep the athlete fresh for the competition attempts. In other words, competition warm-ups will usually be easier than a regular training session because the athlete does not want to risk fatigue at a major competition. If Cao took 22 warm-up sets in the snatch and 18 in the C&J, then we are left with one big question: What do Cao's normal workouts look like when she is not at the Olympics?

The answer is vague because we do not have detailed transcripts of China's workout programs, but we can be absolutely certain that these lifters train with a volume level that fails to comply with any accepted notions of human endurance. Throughout the years, extensive research has been done on the training programs of powerful weightlifting countries such as Bulgaria and the former Soviet Union. We know for a fact that athletes from these countries routinely trained three or four times a day, six days a week, with high intensity percentages at each workout. It stands to reason that China's gradual rise to the top of the world over the last fifteen years has likely been based on this classical Eastern European training methodology. But now that China's success is eclipsing these other traditional power countries, we must acknowledge that they have broken new ground in the training of weightlifters. We can speculate until judgment day about government financial support, drug use, and countless other factors that contribute to their dominance. But the overriding factor of Chinese supremacy is what we can see from Cao Lei's Olympic warm-up progression. Simply put, they're just working a thousand times harder than everybody else.

And now, the training of Mang Foremong...

Now, if the training volume of China's Olympic Champions is one extreme end of the spectrum, the polar opposite end will be an analysis of my own training. Before I go into the details of my training week, it is critical that we admit to some major differences between me and the great lifters of China. For the sake of organization, let's look at it as follows:

- Chinese lifters are in the prime years of their physical abilities. I'm 37

18   **BONES OF IRON**

years old.

- Chinese lifters probably train around 30-40 hours a week. I work around 60 hours a week at my job.
- Chinese lifters have their lives financially subsidized by their government. I have a house payment.
- Chinese lifters spend their non-training time recovering through the use of massage, ice-baths, medical treatment, etc. I spend my non-training time drinking beer and losing my hair.
- Chinese lifters are hand-selected, elite physical specimens. I once tore my groin jumping over a fence.
- Chinese lifters recover from tough workouts quickly because they have more testosterone pumping through their bodies than an 800 lb. Brahma Bull. I'm lifetime drug-free.

The reason why these factors are important is because most of the people who read this article are probably a lot closer to my end of the spectrum. If you're getting older, you work for a living, and you still want to train effectively, then you live in the world I live in (aka, "the real world"). Having said that, here is a complete look at my training routine:

Tuesday	Saturday
- Snatch (light)	- Snatch (heavy)
- Clean and Jerk (light)	- Clean and Jerk (heavy)
- Back Squats (light)	- Back Squat (heavy)

That's it, along with some core work and stretching at the end of each workout. The words "light" and "heavy" are dependent on how close I am to a meet, and I don't use percentages. My current best lifts (within the last year) are 138 kilo snatch, 165 kilo clean and jerk, and 220 kilo back squat. On a typical Tuesday, I will snatch up to 90 kilos for a few singles and C&J up to 120, followed by five or six triples in the back squat up to 175-190 kilos. On a Saturday, I'll usually snatch between 120-130 and C&J around 145-160, followed by squat triples or doubles up to 205-220.

Here are some other pieces of information:

- As I said, I'm 37 years old now. I trained much harder and with much greater volume than this when I was younger. I would not have a 22 year-old lifter use my current workout routine because it's not enough work for a younger lifter. You can handle much more volume when you're in your twenties.
- My selection of exercises (only the snatch, clean and jerk, and back squat) has been determined because of past injuries. Doing pulls and front squats gives me too many problems with my lower back, so I

don't do them anymore. But pulls and front squats were a crucial part of my training when I was younger.

- I train twice a week because that's really all I have time for with my job. Also, I tried going back to three workouts a week last year and I got injured pretty quickly. My recovery time is pretty long now.
- I'm a superheavyweight, usually weighing around 125 kilos (275 lbs.). Heavier lifters have to train with less volume than lighter lifters because their greater mass requires greater recovery time.
- I started training like this in 2007 after a one-year layoff. My total has increased steadily over the last two years, despite increasing age and job demands, and I've had minimal injury trouble.

Okay, so which way do we go?

Now, it's been a lot of fun looking at the volume opposites of these two scenarios, but you've spent this whole article thinking about your own training. You're not a Chinese weightlifter and you're not Matt Foreman, so where is your personal answer? How much volume is right for you? What should your own training program, and the programs of the athletes you coach, look like? Should you train three days a week, five, seven? Should you do four exercises in each workout, two, six? Should you add running, aerobics, swimming, or cycling into your workouts and, if you do, how much is too much?

That's where the art and the science of this business come into play. It is your job, and your challenge, to find the right amount of volume for yourself and the athletes you work with. You will most likely have to consider factors such as job demands, injury history, training experience, motivation level, and a cornucopia of other distractions that will make your job interesting. There will be some trial and error, that's for sure. My advice for newbies would be to get close to somebody who knows much more about training than you do and let them steer the boat for a while. You'll have a few indicators that shine in your face like a police flashlight and they'll tell you if you're getting it right or not. If your athletes' workouts take thirty minutes and none of them are sweating or breathing hard at any time during those thirty minutes, you're probably not planning out enough volume. If your athletes are getting injured regularly and none of them are making any progress in their lifts, you might want to take a look at their workout routine and change something up. If your athletes are making progress and feeling great, then you're on the right track. You might look at a training routine on paper and say to yourself, "This is just too easy. It won't work." But you might be looking at the magic training combination and the only thing that stops you from using it is your desire to be a hard-charging workhorse.

A great track coach once told me, "Motivated athletes will go hard until they're in the hospital, and then rest until they're able to walk again. Lazy athletes will go hard until they see the donut shop, and then rest until their coach yells at them to get working." Since lazy athletes usually just don't hang around weightlifting very long, the chances are that the people you're working with are motivated workers who want to go like hell all the time. Knowing this, your challenge will often be to rein them in before they blow apart. Don't be afraid to pull back when it's obvious that you need to. The amp doesn't have to be set at 11 all the time.

THIRD SNATCH FROM THE SUN

The internet is amazing. It's one of the most important technological developments in the history of modern society, and almost anybody can use it for almost anything. The internet has opened the gates for pure, wonderful experiences such as two old friends reconnecting on Facebook after they lost touch with each other twenty years ago. Likewise, the internet can also be used for evil, immoral purposes such as the perverts we read about in the newspaper who troll around cyberspace looking for victims to abuse.

Somewhere between these two extremes, we have the discussion of lifting weights to get strong. As with everything else, the internet has been the catalyst for miles and miles of discussion on how to get strong and how to be a successful weightlifter. A few days before I sat down to write this article, I decided to check out a few weightlifting message boards and forums because I thought it would be a good way to see what the lifting crowd is talking about the most. In other words, I wanted to direct this month's article at a subject that has been buzzing lately. It probably took me around six or seven minutes to bump into an online conversation about an area that I never get tired of talking about. Apparently, a lot of other people feel the same way.

Here's where I'm going with this. The topic of how to improve Olympic weightlifting performance is endless, and it's not just weightlifters who have their two cents about it. Many powerlifters, and powerlifting coaches, have strong opinions on how our American weightlifters could lift bigger weights and rise back to the top of the world scene. Because they're powerlifters, they usually simplify the whole conversation by going through a soliloquy that sounds something like this: **"American weightlifters just aren't strong enough. They might have solid technique, but they just don't have the squatting and pulling strength to lift the same weights as the Europeans. If Americans wanted to get back to the top of international competition, they need to start putting more emphasis on just getting stronger. And some of the methods used by powerlifters and top powerlifting coaches could accomplish this."**

I wrote these sentences in quotation marks, but they are not a direct quote from anybody. The reason for the quotation marks is that it sounds familiar because we've all heard it before. I've read articles from at least three of America's leading voices in powerlifting that basically say this same thing. The first one I read was in a Muscle and Fitness magazine over twenty years ago, so none of this is new. As you can guess, the Olympic weightlifting community greets these articles with varied responses. Some lifters and coaches believe that there is some merit to the ideas of the powerlifters, and others think that the articles should be used for toilet paper.

And this article is not going to permanently settle anything. Fifty years from now, when Matt Foreman is competing (hopefully) at the National Masters Championships in the 85-89 age group, the iron community will still be arguing about this. The only people who will be listening to me at that point will be the waitresses at Denny's when I blow a gasket because my senior special Grand Slam breakfast was overcharged by four cents.

Here's how we'll do this: I'll throw out a common statement that I've read over and over throughout the years, and then I'll hit it with a double-barrel hot blast of wisdom. This should be sufficient to get some wheels turning and who knows? Maybe this article will make enough sense to somebody that these words eventually get carved into a stone tablet and buried in some kind of lost-ark-of-the-covenant thing which contains all of the universal, irrefutable truths of weightlifting.

I've heard it said many times that "A lot of powerlifters and strongman competitors can power clean and muscle snatch pretty big weights the first time they try it. This is because they're stronger than American Olympic lifters and it means if the Olympic lifters trained like the powerlifters and strongmen, they'd be stronger and more successful. If these powerlifters and strongmen converted to Olympic Lifting full-time, they would dominate."

I know that it is absolutely true that many powerlifters and WSM (world's strongest man) competitors can power clean, power snatch, muscle snatch, etc. pretty impressive weights when they first try them. I can even name a few specific ones. **1)** I personally witnessed world powerlifting champion Bull Stewart power clean 150 kilos in his first workout. The lift looked the way you would imagine; he grabbed the bar, ripped it off the floor, and straight-pulled it to his shoulders like it was an empty bar. **2)** Ed Coan, probably the greatest powerlifter in history, told me in a conversation that he occasionally used power cleans in his training back in his early days and that he had done "four and a quarter for a double" (425 pounds for two reps). Knowing the strength of Ed Coan, I have no problem believing this. **3)** One of the top strongman competitors in the world, Kevin Nee, has a video on YouTube of himself power snatching 130 kilos in training.

All three of these athletes come from a non-Olympic training background and all of them are remarkably strong. Coan has officially deadlifted over 900 pounds at 220 bodyweight, Stewart has done well over 800 at 242, and Nee has competed with the top athletes in the world in the brutal strongman events such as stone lifting and the fingal fingers. With this non-Olympic training background, these men have all been able to dabble with Olympic movements and lift weights that many full-time American Olympic lifters cannot do. With that knowledge, the idea is that if individuals like this converted to Olympic lifting full-time, they would be highly successful at the national and world level. How many American Olympic lifters can power clean 425x2? Probably none, except for maybe the occasional 400 kilo totaler like Shane Hamman or Casey Burgener. And even for them, it would probably be a battle.

Here is something to consider. When a powerlifter or strongman competitor performs the Olympic lifts, they usually use very rough technique. We all know what types of images we're talking about... rounded back, lots of arm pull, no double-knee bend, catching the bar on straight legs. For this article, let's call this "rookie technique." Now, one thing we know for sure is that a superheavyweight weightlifter who wants to compete at the top of the world level will have to snatch around 195 kilos just to be in contention for a medal. Just to compete at the top of the US National level, a superheavyweight will have to snatch around 165 kilos. Keep those numbers in your mind.

There is absolutely nobody on this planet who can snatch 195 kilos with rookie technique. You heard me... nobody. It can't be done. In fact, I would even go so far as to say that there very few athletes anywhere in the world, if any at all, who are strong enough to snatch 165 kilos with rookie technique. To snatch 195 or 165, an athlete has to have a fantastic level of technical skill. The type of technical skill we're talking about can only be developed through intense focus and practice on the actual competition movements of Olympic Weightlifting, the snatch and the clean and jerk. Let's wait until we start turning on NBC every four years and watching the Olympic Games and hearing the commentators saying, "Now walking to the platform is Bob Bronsen. Bob is a powerlifter who convert-ed to Olympic weightlifting two years ago and now he will be attempting a 260 kilo clean and jerk to win the gold medal. Let's watch!" When we hear sound bytes like this, then there might be some merit to the idea that an exceptionally strong athlete from another iron sport could quickly switch to Olympic lifting and rise to the top. The point here is that many of the conversationalists in the strength community speak the belief that converting over to Olympic weightlifting and reaching the top of the mountain is a relatively easy task if the athlete already possesses an ungodly level of pressing, squatting, or strongman-type strength. This is wrong, plain and simple. I saw Shane Hamman compete in his first US national Olympic meet at the 1996 American Open in Savannah, Georgia. Shane snatched 157.5 kilos and got a 175 clean and jerk. He had only been training for a short time before this.

Everyone from every area of the iron game would agree that Shane Ham-man's strength level before he began competing in Olympic lifting was the stuff of legend. An official 1003 squat with strict IPF rules and equipment? Come on, this guy was from another planet. He went on to become the best American superheavyweight ever, eventually totaling 430 kilos. How long did it take one of the strongest squatters in human history to total 430 kilos? Eight years, of full-time concentrated Olympic training. And where did 430 place him at the Olympic Games? Seventh. It just ain't as easy as it looks, Jack.

So let's stay with the dialogue about squatting, Shane, etc. as we get back to our original point. The statement is, **"American Olympic lifters just aren't strong enough to compete with the best lifters in the world."** (That quote will be included in the next issue of *Duh!* Magazine.)

Of course our top US Olympic lifters are not strong enough to compete with the top lifters in the world. This is obvious because **we don't lift as much weight as they do when we compete against them in weightlifting contests**. Nobody is arguing that we aren't as strong as the Europeans and the Chinese. At least nobody should be arguing about it; it's obvious that they're stronger than we are.

BUT... The real question that should be asked is, "How do we develop the specific type of strength that will be necessary to snatch and clean and jerk world-class weights?" That is the Riddle of the Sphinx. And for most of the iron enthusiasts who sermonize this subject on the internet, it all comes down to SQUATTING.

Squatting is the best way to get strong! If you increase your squat strength, you'll snatch and clean more! All the top weightlifters in the world have huge back squats! These are the points that, apparently, every weightlifting coach in America is too stupid to understand. In fact, these points are so important that I think I'll nail one of them individually.

Squatting is the best way to get strong: Yes, squatting is the best way to get strong... at squatting. But is it the best way to get strong at snatching? NO! Now don't get me wrong and think I'm saying that squatting is unimportant for weightlifting success. Squatting, in my opinion, is the most important assistance exercise in weightlifting. But by itself, it will not make you a better snatcher. Snatching does that. I personally went from a 120 snatch to a 135 snatch in one calendar year (April 1993-April 1994). During that same period of time, my back squat increased 2.5 kilos. I would never argue that increasing squat strength is not an important contributor to the development of success in the competition lifts. However, the operative word there is 'contributor.' Squatting is a very important piece of the puzzle in weightlifting, but it is not the only piece.

Let's get back to Shane Hamman and the man who beat him at most of his international competitions, Hossein Rezazedeh. Shane snatched 197.5 kilos and Reza snatched 213. Shane clean and jerked 237.5 kilos and Reza did 263.5. Now, Shane's best powerlifting back squat was 1003 pounds (455 kilos). Reza best back squat was 859 pounds (390 kilos). Shane's 455 was done with powerlifting equipment, granted, and Reza squatted raw. But even squatting raw, Shane could go toe-to-toe with Reza. I have personally seen Shane squat 365 kilos casually after a hard workout with no equipment at all, so hanging with Reza's 390 should be a reasonable assumption. Considering their comparable squatting ability, why could

Reza clean and jerk 26 kilos more than Shane?

The reason is because Reza was stronger than Shane, and Olympic lifting strength is not completely connected to squatting. When an athlete performs snatches, cleans, and jerks, there is a strengthening effect that develops very precisely with the movements. All of the muscles and connective tissues of the body move in a very exact way, and they grow stronger and denser in the positions of the lifts themselves. Every fiber of soft muscle tissue, along with the athlete's tendons and ligaments, increases in strength and power when the athlete performs thousands of snatches or cleans. Bone density even increases in the supportive posture of the lifts. And this type of specific strength takes millions of reps and several years to accumulate. Shane Hamman began practicing the Olympic lifts and strengthening their positions in 1996 when he was twenty-four years old. By any standards, this is a late start. Hossein Rezazedeh began training the Olympic lifts when he was a small child and he had already snatched over 200 kilos when he was twenty-one at the 1999 World Championships. One athlete had a giant head start over the other, end of story. And all the squatting in the world would not be able to change this.

That's the truth, Ruth. But there should be a quick clean-up mentioning of a couple other components in this discussion.

Drugs: Drug use is a subject that applies to every point in this article, but it just isn't the one I'm going to discuss at the moment. Needless to say, every element of weightlifting changes when you start throwing banned performance-enhancing substances into the equation.

Non-Olympic "experts": How should I put this politely? Well, let's look at it this way. I coach football for a living; and every single time I walk out onto the field for a game, there are hundreds of "experts" in the seats right behind me. These are the male fans, mostly fathers of the players, who played football in high school and have never coached a day in their lives. Yet every one of them knows how to coach the team better than me, judging by their comments, and we would all be much more successful if they were calling the plays. You can probably guess how much stock I put in their opinions. This is exactly the way I feel about "experts" who have never coached Olympic Weightlifting but claim that they have the answers to fix our sport in the US. Teaching a man to bench press 800 pounds is not the same as teaching a man to snatch 400 pounds. It might seem like the same idea and there might even be some common ground between the two, but they just aren't the same thing. Perhaps the best way to put a cherry on top of this is to say that some people are simply more talented at certain things than others. Nobody ever taught Jimi Hendrix to play the guitar the way he did. Jackson Pollack didn't learn his "drip technique" from attending a painting seminar. Both of these men achieved greatness in their fields because they were born with something special that nobody else had. But Jimi didn't perfect the guitar by playing the violin all day and Jackson didn't create masterpiece paintings by spending years drawing crayon pictures. They focused on their specific medium until they eventually broke new ground and created works of art that seemed more like they were dropped onto this planet from an alternate universe. This is what athletes have to do if they want to break new ground with the snatch and the clean and jerk. Is weightlifting success as simple as this? It's as simple as standing next to a mountain and chopping it down with the edge of your hand.

BOMBING

The first really big weightlifting meet I competed in was the 1994 US Olympic Festival. You had to be specially selected to compete in this meet, and it was an all-expenses paid trip to lift with the best in the country. It was a huge deal. I got picked to lift that year, and I showed up in the best shape of my life. In the competition, I missed all three of my snatches and bombed out of the contest. It was the worst moment of my life up to that point. As I walked back into the warm-up room after I bombed, I saw weightlifting legend Mario Martinez standing there. Mario was also competing in this meet and he was getting ready to start warming up for his own snatch attempts. Mario was a legend, as I said, and I walked over to him and asked, "Hey Mario, have you ever bombed out of a big meet?" I had never met him and he didn't know who I was, but he was very cool to me. He said, "Yeah, a few times. It happens, just keep your head up." It made me feel great to hear him say that. Then, about ten minutes later, Mario went out there and missed all three of his snatches, also bombing out of the contest. I was pretty sure he was going to punch me in the face for jinxing him, but he didn't. I'm glad, because it would have hurt really bad.

THE SNATCH
ALSO RISES

Ernest Hemingway is my favorite writer of all time. His personal life was almost as legendary as the books he wrote, filled with great victories and plenty of sad moments as well. When he won the Nobel Prize in Literature in 1954, he was still enjoying the success of his novel *The Old Man and the Sea,* although his health and mental condition had already started a slow descent. Right around this time period, an interviewer asked Hemingway, "What is the best early training for a writer?" This was a terrific question and it gave the world a chance to hear something valuable from the master. Ernest's answer was, "An unhappy childhood."

If that sounds difficult to understand, read a book about Hemingway's life (preferably the one written by Carlos Baker) and it will all make sense after a while. And if you're patiently waiting for this particular article to actually start talking about strength training and weightlifting, I'll oblige you now. Ernest's quote about early training for a writer makes me think about lifting. Specifically, it makes me think about the physical and mental qualities that can identify someone as a potentially successful weightlifter. What are the things that a coach can look for that will function as early predictors of high weightlifting ability? Are there specific combinations of athleticism, flexibility, body structure, etc. that can give us an accurate idea about whether or not an individual might become a national champion in the snatch and clean and jerk? In other words, what should a coach look for in a potential trainee? What are the attributes that should make you approach a gym rat and ask if he/she has any interest in learning how to be a weightlifter?

I'll give you four of them. Ernest was married four times, so the number seems appropriate.

To Jump and Jump Not

Many of the top international weightlifting programs of the last thirty years have used jumping ability as one of the absolute highest determinants of weightlifting potential. If an athlete has natural jumping ability, then that athlete already has a large advantage in the sport of weightlifting (and most other sports, actually). This ability can be measured in a variety of ways. The standing long jump, standing vertical jump measured by a Vertec jump measurement, box jumping for height, and a variety of other testing methods will give an immediate indication of the athlete's explosive power and potential lower body strength. Now, when a 6'5 basketball player can dunk on a ten-foot rim with approach steps, this can be misleading. When I was a strength and conditioning coach at Northern Arizona University in the early 90s, many of our basketball players were shocked to find out that their vertical jumps only measured around 28-30 inches on a Vertec. These players were all over 6'5 and they could perform all kinds of acrobatic dunks on the court, but their vertical jump measurements were relatively un-impressive. Their dunking ability was mostly related to their height, arm length, and run-up acceleration into takeoff of the dunk. Most of the top vertical jump numbers came from the sprinters and throwers on the track team, as they often possessed much greater explosive power in the lower body.

The reason for the close connection between jumping ability and weightlift-ing success is the jump-like movement that takes place in the pulling phase of the snatch and clean. When an athlete is completing the pull of the Olympic lifts, the mechanics of the body are very similar to the mechanics of a standing vertical jump and, obviously, explosive force is essential in both activities. Now, if you read a lot of weightlifting message boards on the internet, you'll know that many coaches are perpetually engaged in a biblical war of annihilation over the proper terminology to describe the pulling movement of the snatch and clean. Some coaches want to refer to it as a "jumping motion." Some coaches want to refer to it as a "catapult motion." On and on it goes, and almost nobody ever agrees on anything. But regardless of whether you want to refer to the pulling motion as a jump, catapult, ricochet, crossbow, slingshot, uppercut, jump-down-turn-around-pick-a-bale-of-cotton, or whatever, it is clear that jumping power is a valuable weapon to the Olympic lifter. I once taught a high school weightlifting class and one of the students was a sixteen year-old young man who was approximately 5'7 and 160 pounds. He was a skateboarder, borderline juvenile delinquent, and a very clear candidate for the Most Likely to Get Kicked in the Head Award. But he was naturally springy, he could nail a standing backflip at any moment, and he thought weightlifting looked cool. So after a few recruiting speeches and a few threats, I convinced him to give lifting a shot. Two years later, he went to the Junior National Championships and made a 102.5 snatch and 137.5 clean and jerk in the 77 kilo class.

There are countless other examples in our sport just like this. Shane Hamman could do backflips. Many of our top female weightlifters have gymnastics backgrounds. Nicu Vlad had one of the highest tested vertical jumps at the Olympic Training Center. The list goes on. If you want to find out if you've got a potential stud on your hands, start with the hops, homie.

The Torrents of Stretching

So... the kid can jump. He can do snappy round-offs and a ten-foot standing long

BONES OF IRON

jump and he can get on top of a 48-inch box. Great! Now, we need to find out about flexibility.

Any exposure at all to Olympic Weightlifting will make it obvious that good flexibility is mandatory. However, weightlifting flexibility is somewhat specific. When most people think about flexibility, they tend to look at general positions that are commonly regarded as strong indicators. Can the athlete do the splits and get all the way down to the floor? Can the athlete do a back bridge and get the hands close to the feet? Can the athlete get on his/her knees and bend backwards until the head touches the floor? These are great positional tests and they can certainly make it clear how limber the person is.

But "weightlifting flexibility" is measured in a much simpler way. How flexible is the athlete in the actual positions of the snatch, clean, and jerk? For example, let's say you have a young woman who can do the splits. That's terrific. But it's more important in weightlifting to find out how flexible she is in a deep squat position. Can she sit down into a full squat and demonstrate all the important elements? In other words, can she sit her hamstrings and butt down on her calves, keep her heels flat on the floor, and push her knees forward with her torso upright? This is the absolute most important measure of flexibility in Olympic Weightlifting, and many people tip over like a drunk on payday when they try it for the first time. Other flexibility tests are interesting and they have their place in basic physical assessment, but the full-squat test is absolutely Numero Uno if we're talking about the Olympic lifts.

After the squatting flexibility has been determined, the second most important area is the positions of the shoulders and elbows. To put it more simply, we're talking about lockout. When you (the coach) start working with a potential trainee, one of the first things that need to happen is an overhead lockout with a broomstick or empty bar. You have to know right away if the athlete has straight, bone-on-bone lockout. If those elbows straighten out naturally and that bar looks like it's being supported effortlessly by the athlete's skeletal structure with a nice wide chest position, then you know you're in business. If the athlete extends the empty bar overhead and you're looking at the chicken-wing crooked lockout that we've all seen at some point, then it's clear that you've got your work cut out for you.

I was talking to longtime US coach Roger Nielson once and he told me that he remembered the first workout of Jeff Michels, who went on to become one of the strongest American lifters of all time with a 188 kilo snatch and 222.5 kilo clean and jerk in the old 110 kilo weight class. Jeff began lifting when he was very young and I asked Roger, "Could you tell that Jeff was going to be great when you saw his first workout?" Roger told me that it was obvious Jeff "had something special" because he was able to sit down in the bottom position of a snatch with a bar over his head and it looked like he was born there. If you ever get a chance to see any footage of Jeff's top lifts, you'll see what Roger meant. His natural level of weightlifting flexibility put him miles ahead of his peers from day one.

Video Games and the Collapse of American Masculinity

I think that sounds like a great title for a book, don't you? It sounds a little gender-specific, but let me explain where I'm going for the men and the ladies too. When a coach examines a potential lifter, I think one of the most valuable traits to look for is the evidence of some general physicality. In other words, you want to see people who have had some kind of vigorous bodily development in their background. I'll give you a personal example of what I'm talking about. My father was a rugged, old-school coal miner from Kentucky who refused to let his sons grow up soft and weak. From the earliest days of my memory, my brother and I were required to be involved in some kind of physically taxing activity. This usually came from the work we had to do around the house. Spending our afternoons in the backyard swinging a heavy axe over and over while we split firewood, turning wrenches while we helped him work on our cars and home repairs, digging ditches in our yard to install a sprinkler system, things like that. We weren't allowed to sit inside all day and play Call of Duty. Our job was to complete the grunt work of our family and when we had free time to play, we jumped on our BWX bikes and pedaled like maniacs or we went to our friends' houses to wrestle and pound the crap out of each other. To put it simply, most of our childhood involved hard work, even if we were playing. By the time we got old enough to join sports teams at school, we were already used to sweating and getting sore.

And we all know that our society has changed as technology has accelerated. These days, the internet and Sony Playstation have given our youth plenty of opportunities to grow up on the couch. In many cases, young kids can reach their teenage years with virtually no evidence of any kind of development in their muscles or skeletal system. Not to mention the fact that they've lived on a steady diet of Cheetos and chicken nuggets since birth. Hard to imagine that we're not churning out armies of Jim Thorpes, isn't it? These kids fracture their wrists when they trip on the sidewalk because their bones are squishy little columns of pus. Well, before I turn this into a long-winded rant on the laziness of today's youth, I'll get back to the point. Young people (or people of any age) are going to have an easier learning curve in weightlifting if they come to the sport with some form of GPP (General Physical Preparedness). If you've done any coaching, you know that it's extremely easy to see which athletes have some kind of physical background and which ones have none. Weightlifting is a very, very tough sport. Some evidence of core development, connective tissue strength, and bone density are going to help the early training days dramatically, regardless of where these traits were developed.

And finally...

What kind of mental attributes will make a successful weightlifter?

This question really deserves its own article, because the answer could be analyzed endlessly. Most people who have trained or competed in Olympic Weight-lifting for a substantial length of time will tell you that the mental challenge of weightlifting is just as severe as the physical. As a twenty-two year competitor in the sport, I can honestly say that weightlifting has tested every possible area of my mind, soul, and personality. The ability to overcome pain is essential. You're going to hurt in this sport, plain and simple. The willingness to make a long-term commitment to your goals is mandatory. You say you want to compete in the Olympic Trials, right? What if it's going to take eight years of your life to get there? Now what? The determination to revolve your life around your training is demanded. How many parties are you willing to pass up and how many relationships are you willing to terminate if they are stopping you from reaching your goals?

These are extreme questions, and not every potential trainee is going to be interested in making a complete, fanatical commitment to weightlifting. Some people just want to work out and the Olympic lifts seem like a fun way to do it. That's fine. But regardless, there are still certain mental qualities that will make the athletes much more successful if they have them. Let's put down a list:

- Detail-oriented
- Enjoys constant repetition of the same skill
- Ability to be patient and impatient at the same time
- Willingness to overcome fear
- Internally motivated
- Competitive
- Doesn't blame others for failure
- Hates whining
- Respects authority
- Enjoys hard work

The presence of each of these, along with some of the physical attributes we've examined, are the building blocks of a champion. But there is one more truth to reveal, and it's probably the biggest one in the weightlifting universe. It's the seminal element of weightlifting training, both as a competitive sport and a recreational pursuit. It's the most crucial concept in this sport.

And here it is...

Some athletes have tremendous physical talent and outstanding mental ability. These are the ones that make Olympic teams. As a coach, you'll get an athlete like this every once in a great while (if ever). The vast majority of the athletes you coach will be people who have a few great qualities and several mediocre ones. You'll work with some athletes who have phenomenal jumping ability, but they're mental midgets. You'll work with some athletes who are incredibly dedicated and focused, but they couldn't jump over a speed bump if they were shot out of a rocket launcher. You'll work with some athletes who have perfect flexibility and body proportions, but they don't really care that much if they make progress in their lifts. You'll work with athletes who have more natural strength in their first training session than the five-year veterans in your gym, but their emotional problems make them almost impossible to tolerate.

Whatever assortment of positives and negatives the athlete brings to the table, the great coaches are the ones who can always find a way to make people better. The strong kid with the intolerable attitude? A great coach will find a way to develop that kid. The focused athlete with low physical talent? A great coach will find a way to develop that person. The ex-gymnast girl who is built perfectly for the sport but cries every single day in the gym? A great coach will find a way to develop that girl. Great coaches have to possess a fantastic proficiency in lifting technique and program design, but they also need to have the ability to manage every imaginable kind of personality while still maintaining the integrity of their program. Are there times when it's appropriate to kick someone out of your gym? Absolutely. But those cases are extremely rare, in my experience.

If an athlete has very low physical ability but is willing to stick to it for a long period of time, that athlete will eventually be successful. Remember that if you remember nothing else. Hard times and frustration are guaranteed, but they can be overcome. As Ernest himself once wrote, "The world breaks everyone and afterward many are strong in the broken places." Figure that quote out, and you've figured out weightlifting.

BO KNOWS POWER CLEANS: CROSS-TRAINING AND OLYMPIC WEIGHTLIFTING

These days, you're showing your age when you talk about the exploits of Bo Jackson. For those of you who don't remember (in other words, those of you who weren't around in the eighties), Bo Jackson was an athletic phenomenon of galactic proportions. As an All-Star major league baseball player with the Kansas City Royals, Bo was a fearsome hitter who could smash home runs into the opposite hemisphere. As an NFL running back with the Los Angeles Raiders, Bo was a wrecking machine who could simultaneously score touchdowns and humiliate linebackers like Brian Bosworth by running over them like they were Girl Scouts. Bo was a professional two-sport athlete, and it didn't take long for the Nike corporation to build a marketing campaign around him.

Bo became a poster child for the idea of "cross training." I put that term in quotation marks because, back in the eighties, it was a revolutionary concept. Being able to use a variety of sports training methods to become a strong overall athlete was the theory behind cross training. Nike made commercials that showed Bo Jackson playing football, baseball, basketball, running, lifting weights, etc. All of this, of course, was a business strategy for Nike to sell their hot line of Cross Training shoes. But it didn't take long for the fitness industry to buy into the concept of cross training and now, twenty years later, the practice of using multiple training disciplines to build well-rounded athleticism is one of the fundamental principles of the workout world.

Knowing this, it quickly becomes clear that there has to be some common sense used in the planning of cross training. This is especially important if the athlete in question is focusing some, most, or all of their efforts on Olympic weightlifting. Organizations such as Catalyst Athletics have chosen to use the Olympic lifts as part of the foundation of their training approach because most athletes and trainers with brains in their heads have figured out that the Olympic lifts are incredibly effective tools for developing overall strength and athleticism. However, many coaches and lifters have posed a common question over the years, "What are some non-Olympic lifting exercises that can help develop the Olympic lifts?" Are there other training activities aside from the snatch and clean and jerk that can contribute to the athlete's improvement? And, conversely, are there any exercises that could act as setbacks to the Olympic lifts, damaging the athlete's progress in the snatch or clean and jerk?

We can end the suspense by stating a few basic truths from the stone commandment tablets of weightlifting scripture. First, your training should be completely focused on the Olympic lifts if you want to be a good Olympic weightlifter. If being an Olympic lifter is not your primary focus, then branching out and exploring new training styles should be the fundamental guide for your regimen. Second, there are non-Olympic exercises that can provide some benefit to the weightlifter and, likewise, there are non-Olympic exercises that can harm the weightlifter's progress. What we will do in this article is take a close look at five popular training activities and how each one of them can have a positive or negative effect on the training of a weightlifter. This information should be equally useful for serious Olympic weightlifting coaches and also for general strength training athletes who use the Olympic lifts in their workouts.

Running

Let's just get the biggest one out of the way first. Running is one of the most popular forms of exercise in the world. The health benefits of running are well documented and they don't need to be covered here. There are also potential injuries, such as stress fractures and plantar fasciaitis, that can occur from running. Over the years, I have heard the question thrown out on many occasions. "Should running be a part of an Olympic lifter's training?"

The first thing I want to say about this is that I've been an Olympic lifter for over twenty years and it has been my good fortune to train with some of the best weightlifters in the world. I have never seen a high-quality Olympic lifter who used running as any significant part of their training. I once trained with a national champion who decided to drop to a lower weight class, and he incorporated some running workouts into his training week to lose bodyweight. I have also seen a few elite lifters who have spent very brief periods running short sprints or hill workouts in an effort to build explosiveness. But none of these athletes used running for very long and most of them confined it to very short sprint work. Running will provide some extra pounding on the joints of the lower body, it will often reduce the athlete's bodyweight, and it will sap away at least a small portion of the athlete's energy supply. All of these risk factors can be easily justified if the athlete is a basic cross trainer, but they are difficult to justify if the athlete is training for the highest possible results in weightlifting competition. When I was doing the best lifting of my career, I did absolutely no running whatsoever. However, I will also say that if I were not a competitive weightlifter, I would definitely include it as part of my training.

Tire Flipping

This one has gained tremendous popularity over the last ten years. When I was in high school, the only place you saw massive diesel truck tires being flipped was on the practice fields of football teams. Then, people started watching the World's Strongest Man contests on ESPN and they couldn't believe how cool it was to see some rhinoceros named Gunther blasting these massive tires up and down a runway. Nowadays, soccer moms have them in their back yards next to the trampoline so they can get a good workout before their next pedicure/botox appointment. The majority of fitness trainers in the industry like to use tire flipping with their clients. The strength-building benefits can, in theory, provide assistance to competitive weightlifters. Tire flipping is an excellent activity for building grip strength. The forearms and hands will usually be screaming after a dozen flips with a challenging tire. The core strengthening involved in tires is considerable as well, and core strengthening is a universal positive for any weightlifter, athlete, or human being who wants to live well. If there is any negative for Olympic lifters, it would basically be the same one we discussed in running. Tire flipping, at least as it's done by most trainers, involves some endurance. Endurance equals sweating and breathing hard, which equals burning calories, which equals loss of bodyweight. Loss of bodyweight is almost always a detriment for a competitive Olympic weightlifter.

Strongman Activity

Along the same lines with tire flipping, strongman training has grown in popularity over the last twenty years mainly because of ESPN's coverage of the WSM. These days, whenever I tell civilians that I'm an Olympic weightlifter, one of the first things that usually comes out of their mouths is, "Do you do that strongman stuff like the guys on ESPN?" Because of the rise in popularity, some of the events from strongman have caught on with the general strength training crowd. Several barbell supply companies now sell the large metal cylinders that are used to practice the log lift. Stone loading is gradually starting to catch on, although this one is difficult because of how rare the equipment is. But these two examples are good ones to take a look at. How would stone loading and log lifting have a positive or negative effect on the Olympic lifts?

Positively, it is clear that these two events, along with many of the other strongman events, teach the athlete to use the body in a technical way, much the same as the snatch or clean and jerk. Stone loading involves taking a heavy object from the floor using the back, legs, shoulders, hips, etc. Sound familiar? The log lift is actually somewhat modeled after the clean and jerk. When athletes perform these strength feats, they are learning the concept of coordinating each body part together into one fluid movement. There is some carryover to the Olympic lifts here because of the obvious basic similarity in ideas. In other words, you learn stone loading technique just like you learn snatch technique. This is a positive carryover, in addition to the fact that strongman events like the ones mentioned here are guaranteed to develop greater back and grip strength.

If there is a negative to using the strongman events in combination with the Olympic lifts, it would simply be that the strongman events are incredibly demanding in their physicality. If an athlete heads to the gym to do a heavy snatch workout twenty-four hours after a hard session of stone loading, the fatigue in the muscles of the back would be considerable. For that matter, most of the strongman events would need to be worked into an Olympic lifter's training regimen very carefully because of the extra soreness that would follow. When an athlete is pushing the limits of their capability in the Olympic lifts, the body has to be primed and ready in order to be successful. If you've ever gone to the gym with back muscles that feel like you gave Jabba the Hut a piggyback ride and then tried to hit some heavy snatches, you understand what I mean.

Martial Arts Training

Here we have an interesting analysis because martial arts training is the only activity mentioned so far that has a direct combative element to it. In running, tire flipping, or strongman activity, there is always some predictability. You basically know exactly what the ground, the tire, or the stones are going to do at all times (unless you're jogging in a mine field). But in martial arts training, when an athlete is sparring or grappling with another athlete, there is a certain degree of uncertainty. The athlete you are grappling with might decide to roll you over and put you in a guillotine choke hold, an ankle lock, or dozens of other possible positions. All of these positions have the potential to hurt you.

Now that mixed martial arts (UFC) has become one of the most popular sports on the planet, the client demand for training is on the rise. If an athlete wants to train the Olympic lifts seriously but also wants to incorporate some kind of martial arts training into their program, there can be both positives and negatives. I personally think one of the biggest benefits to martial arts training is the mental toughness and fearlessness that develops in the athlete's mind. I was a wrestler in high school, and I still think of my wrestling practices as some of the most physically demanding experiences of my life. To borrow a phrase from wrestling legend Dan Gable, everything else seems easy after you've been a wrestler. Also, martial arts training teaches an athlete not to shy away from anything. Having to step onto a mat with another human being and literally fight to keep from being defeated is a powerful source of energy. The athlete simply stops being scared of anything, and the connection to the Olympic lifts is huge in this department because a certain degree of fearlessness is required to be a good weightlifter.

Are there any negatives to incorporating martial arts training into a weightlifting regimen? The one that comes to mind quickly is injury. I have personally trained with two good weightlifters who had their elbow lockout permanently damaged through grappling. Their opponents used arm bar submission holds on them and cranked too hard, and some long-term joint damage was the result. Their ability to lock out their snatches and jerks was never the same afterwards. Obviously, this type of injury isn't going to happen to everyone who trains in the martial arts, but you get the idea. It's hard to have a good clean and jerk workout the day after somebody kicks you in the face and breaks your nose.

Bodybuilding

I know, I know... but just wait a minute. Most of the die-hard weightlifters I've met in my life exhibit a type of cringing nausea reaction when you say the word "bodybuilding" to them. Their faces usually look like they just smelled cat urine. But let's not throw the baby out with the banana peels. Can we at least admit that there are some good things about bodybuilding? First of all, absolutely everybody on this planet thinks it's cool to have great looking pecs, calves, and biceps. Second, bodybuilders have a lot of good things to teach us about how to develop a sound training diet. Third, bodybuilders spend their days constantly thinking about barbells. How bad can they be? But the important question here is, "If an athlete wants to incorporate Olympic weightlifting into bodybuilding training, will there be any benefits or hazards?"

Benefits: There will be some strength gains. Even if an athlete performs bodybuilding-style movements and uses high repetitions, the training will develop strength. Make no mistake about it, there are some very strong bodybuilders out there. Granted, most of them are taking enough drugs to blast the next space shuttle into orbit. But even the bodybuilders who train naturally are able to pack on some solid muscle and move some respectable iron.

Hazards: Bodybuilding training generally focuses on slow, controlled movements. Weightlifting depends on fast, controlled movements. Bodybuilding exercises are designed to isolate certain body parts and train them one at a time. Weightlifting requires the athlete to use all body parts together at the same time. No offense meant to our spandex speedo brothers and sisters, but bodybuilding doesn't require a high degree of athleticism (agility, coordination, balance, explosiveness, etc.). Weightlifting is completely dependent on athleticism. Bodybuilding's ultimate goal is physical appearance. Physical appearance has nothing to do with weightlifting success. The main idea here is that these two styles of training are diametrically opposed. There just isn't much carryover between them.

In an alternate universe...

All of these training activities, along with several others, are major points of interest for athletic enthusiasts. When an athlete has trained in one specific way for a long period of time, boredom can start to set in. Even if the athlete loves what they do, the occasional itch to do something new will pop up. For example, I've been an Olympic weightlifter for most of my life and I love it more than anything in the world. However, I also have the personality type to look at other athletic skills and say, "Hey, it would be cool to do that!" A few years ago, I started competing in the Scottish Highland Games and I've had a blast doing it. Being a weightlifter has given me a good strength base for throwing and the contests themselves are a total hoot. However, training for the games is demanding and it involves a lot of wear and tear on the body. I've had to seriously curtail my enthusiasm for throwing because the physical exertion of it takes a toll on my training as a weightlifter.

I used that example to illustrate the point that any activity you do is going to affect all the other ones. Running is going to have an impact on your lifting. Lifting is going to have an impact on your running. Etcetera, etcetera... If you make the decision to combine multiple training disciplines, there has to be a sensible plan involved. Unfortunately, that plan will probably require a lot of trial and error to master. You might not find out just how much stone loading is too much until you strain one of your rhomboids. You might be having a ball doing bodybuilding bicep workouts until you start to notice that you're having trouble locking out your jerks over your head. Every athlete has limits and the human body can only withstand a certain amount of labor. Just ask Bo Jackson, whose brilliant career was eventually ended by injury. He went from being a two-sport superstar to being a retired two-sport superstar with plenty of time to go fishing. Trying to fish with multiple poles at once is a tricky business. You'd better know what you're going to do if each pole hooks a fish at the same moment.

International Olympic Committee founder Pierre de Coubertin once said, "All sports for all people." But I have it on good authority that he was a lousy snatcher. Choose wisely, mon amis.

STUPIDITY

A friend of mine once snatched 120 kilos (264 pounds) with no warm-up. He just walked up to the bar and snatched it, didn't even do any stretching first. We had been in a bar drinking for five or six hours and we remembered a story we heard where Soviet Olympic Champion David Rigert once snatched 170 kilos (374 pounds) with no warm-up. If you know anything about David Rigert, you believe this story. There were a bunch of eyewitnesses anyway. My friend said he could snatch 120 the same way, no warm-up, stretching, or preparation. His best snatch ever at the time was around 140 kilos, so 120 was a big lift for him. We left the bar and went to the gym. It was around 1:00 am, we were quite drunk, wearing street clothes and running shoes. We loaded 120 on the bar and he snatched it. It was fun. My coach back in those days used to get pissed off at my friend and me because he said we did too much stupid stuff that messed up our training. I don't know why he thought that.

CONTROLLING THE TORNADO: PLANNING YOUR TRAINING, PART ONE

This article will be focused on planning out your training program. And you're out of your mind if you think I'm going to start with a slogan that you've already heard a million times like "Failing to plan is planning to fail." This slogan is a proven truth, but it should be painfully obvious. I shouldn't have to remind you that planning is important any more than I should have to remind you not to eat yellow snow.

However, there is obviously a good reason why slogans like this are used so often. Most people understand that having a solid plan of attack before beginning any endeavor is going to put you in a much better position to be successful. When we listen to interviews with people who have been highly accomplished in their fields, whether the field is athletics or business, one of the most common aspects of their achievements is precise planning. I can't remember ever reading an article about an Olympic gold medalist where the athlete said, "For my workouts, I just kinda come to the gym and do whatever I feel like doing that day." Bill Gates never told the world, "I just hired some people to help me make computers. I don't know how the hell my company grew so much." Nope, sorry. Elite personalities usually approach things from the opposite direction.

Take Lance Armstrong, for example. This guy won seven Tour de France races while pedaling with only one testicle. I once read that one of Armstrong's nicknames is "Mr. Millimeter." People started calling Lance by this name because of his obsessive, fanatical attention to proper preparation. In all aspects of his training and performance, Armstrong analyzes and refines every single detail down to razor-sharp perfection. In a sport like Olympic weightlifting, these personalities are just as prevalent. I once saw a documentary on the Bulgarian weightlifting program of the 1980s where coach Ivan Abadjiev was in a shouting match with superheavyweight world champion Antonio Krastev. Krastev wanted to snatch 200 kilos in a particular workout, and Abadjiev's training plan had dictated that Krastev would only be able to snatch 195 that day. The film showed Krastev taking multiple attempts at 200 and barking at Abadjiev, "I can do 200!" Abadjiev watched and continued to admonish Antonio with, "No, you will not do a gram more than 195 today." Like Lance Armstrong, Abadjiev put amazing amounts of time and concentration into his training plans.

Because of all these examples and because of the importance of this topic, this article will be the first in a three-part series. This month, we will examine the planning of yearly training. Next month, we will focus on the preparation of individual training cycles within a given year. And then the series will conclude with a third article about the planning of individual workouts within those training cycles. Sounds organized, huh? Hey, you get high quality here at the Performance Menu.

365 days. What to do?

Although these articles are obviously focused on Olympic Weightlifting, there are plenty of valuable concepts to be discussed that are equally applicable to generalized Crossfit training, fighting, cycling, bodybuilding, or any other discipline where progress is expected.

When looking at a year of competition and training, the first step on the road is goal analysis. Ask yourself what you want to accomplish in 2010 or any other year you're approaching. Weightlifting is a very easy sport to set goals in because the sport is centered on numbers. If your best competition lifts are a 100 kilo snatch and 130 kilo clean and jerk, you might decide that 10 kilos of progress in each lift during a full year is reasonable. However, there are several variables to factor into this phase of your goal setting. For example, let's say that your best competition lifts are 100/130, but you are a 120 kilo man who only trained two months to achieve those lifts, your technique is improving, and your base strength level is through the roof (legitimate 500 pound squat, 550 deadlift, etc.) In this case, ten kilos of improvement on each lift in one year might be too conservative. For this hypothetical athlete, I would not hesitate to expect around 120/150 or more after a full year of concentrated training.

Then, let's look at another example. In this situation, the athlete has best competition lifts of 100/130 but the lifter is an elite female national champion in the 75 kilo class who has been training full-time for ten years and holds all the American records. With this lifter, planning for 110/140 in one year might be a bit of a stretch. The point is that all of these details factor into the setting of goals. And to complicate things even more, it must be acknowledged that most people will have to work around several "distraction factors" when they plan out their competition year. What are distraction factors? Here are two of the biggest ones:

Work: Do you have a job that will make training or competing difficult/impossible at certain times during the year? Military, traveling salesman, etc. These professions can alter your competitive year. For a personal example, I'm a masters weightlifter and my current totals are good enough to qualify for the masters world championships. However, I'm also a high school football coach, and the masters world championship is held right smack in the middle of football season every year (October-November). Because of this, I can't plan to attend the masters worlds unless I'm willing to lose my job. This, my friends, is a distraction factor. Jobs are wonderful at throwing wrenches into your machinery.

Family: No, I'm not classifying your family as a distraction. But if you're married and have children, there will be certain responsibilities that you have to account for. For example, they will probably want to take a vacation every year; and your vacation time will probably not center around you finding a gym close to Disneyland so you can train while your screaming kids get strapped into Space Mountain... alone... and your spouse thumbs through the Holiday Inn yellow pages for a good divorce lawyer. If you want to take a family vacation in the summer and you also want to compete in weightlifting meets, you will have to coordinate these things in a way that will provide both maximum performance and big family fun.

Your life has its own challenges. The important idea here is that you have to try to cover all the bases when you are planning out your training. Think of everything. All of the real-life obstacles that can potentially surface have to be added into your plan. Do you live in an area where there aren't many weightlifting meets to compete in during the year? If so, you will have to travel when you want to compete. Where will your finances allow you to travel to, and how often? These elements all matter, and you have a much better shot at being successful if you have all of the land mines located before you start walking through the field.

One more thing: There might be some of you who have no distraction factors in your life. You're not married yet, you don't have a real job or you're still going to school, etc. If this is your situation and the only thing you really have to think about in life is your training, then more power to you. You're living in that short window of life when you basically get to be a full-time athlete and nothing else matters. That's a special time, believe me, and you'd better enjoy it while it lasts. But his article is focused more on athletes and coaches who have entered the "real world" stage of life and have to juggle their training with mortgage payments, deadlines, day care, and every other speed bump that gets thrown in the road.

Meets, meets, meets...

Most successful weightlifters have a fairly specific idea of what their competition schedule will look like each year. There are three primary questions to answer when planning out a competitive year:

1. How many meets do you want to compete in during the year?

2. How far apart are these meets and how much training time will you have for each one?

3. Which meets are most important to you?

Now, the considerations that go into each one:

How many? Weightlifting is much different from sports like track and field, soccer, and baseball where the athlete can compete every weekend or twice a week. The average weightlifter will usually compete five or six times per year. If the athlete plans to compete more often than this, most of the competitions will likely be "training meets." A training meet is where the athlete lifts in a competition but deliberately takes conservative attempts with weights that are roughly the same as the athlete's average workout. This allows the athlete to compete often without the physical demands of "peaking" for each contest. I would not advise a competition schedule where the athlete is planning to lift in eight meets per year and peak for each one. The risk of injury is high with a schedule like this. The exception would be young beginners who are lifting weights that are well within their total body strength level and have lightning-fast recovery time. These athletes can, and should, compete often. But as the athlete ages, the recovery time demands will grow.

How far apart? More important meets will generally require more preparation time, and training meets require very little. If an athlete is planning to compete in a national championship, 10-12 weeks of uninterrupted training would probably provide a solid base that builds up to a sharp peak at the end. Some athletes prefer more time than this, and others can perform well with less. If an athlete is planning to compete in Jethro's Weightliftin' Bonanza where the meet will be held in a barn and the awards are shots of Jager, 10-12 weeks of preparation probably won't be necessary.

Most important? This is based on your performance level. The top of your mountain might be the state, national, or world championship. If you are a national champion, the state championship will likely be a training meet. If you have no realistic chance of qualifying for a national contest, the state championship could be your big peak of the year. Regardless of your skill and competitive ranking, it is imperative that you decide which competition you want to achieve your maximum results at. I have seen several athletes over the years who hit their biggest numbers at the wrong time. For example, world team members should clearly register their biggest totals of the year at the world championship. If the athlete lifts fantastic weights at the national championship and then goes on to perform a 10-15 kilo decrease at the world championship three months later, something was wrong with the athlete's preparation plan (unless he/she was battling other setbacks such as injury or illness).

Here is a basic outline of what many of our top Calpian weightlifters did on a yearly basis during the 1990s in Washington:

- February: Oregon Cup Championship (training meet)
- April/May: Senior National Championship (peak meet)
- June: Oregon Classic (training meet)
- August: The Bad Mother Open (training meet, and I should write an article about this one some day)
- October: Washington Open (training meet)
- December: American Open (peak meet)

This was a common plan for our club lifters, but there were obviously some variations. In the 90s, we usually had two or three lifters in our gym who were world team members. They would often skip some of the training meets, such as the Washington Open in October, to get more preparation time for the world championship. We also had lifters who competed in other national meets such as the junior or collegiate nationals. These types of meets would obviously add another peak performance into the competition year and probably require the dropping of a training meet somewhere. However, it is worth adding that our Calpian athletes trained at a very high level throughout the year. Most of the lifters in our club were capable of lifting weights that were within a few kilos of their personal records on a regular basis, and this made peaking three or four times a year much easier. We trained very hard and we were ready to load up the bar at the drop of a hat.

DOWN time...

I can make this one quick and easy. Plan some light recovery time into your training year, preferably immediately after peak competitions. Your results will be much better and your body will last longer if you back off the heavy training for a while after major contests. What is "down time" exactly?

Down time might involve staying away from the barbell for a short time. Older lifters would be especially wise to consider this. Training hard and peaking for a big contest when you're 30-40-50+ years old is extremely taxing on the body. After a major contest, there is nothing wrong with a week of stretching, core work, and some other non-barbell activity such as swimming. That week can be followed by another week or two of "transition lifting," where you head back to the gym but you spend time doing variety exercises that are different from your normal routine. Kettlebells are excellent at this point. After this week, it will be time to go back to the barbell and start working the competition movements again as you begin the new cycle for your next competition.

For you twenty-four year-olds, you don't get off as easy. "Down time" for a younger lifter after a major peak competition will usually be shorter (three or four days) and the return to the competition lifts will be quick, although the percentages will obviously be lighter as the athlete's physiology recovers from the strain of the contest. Some coaches choose to have their athletes do nothing but pulls and squats for two weeks following a major contest. This type of work keeps the athlete from losing strength but also gives the joints (and the brain) a rest from the heavy snatches and jerks.

And once you've taken a look at all of these elements and also attempted to plan out every other aspect of your life, you're ready to put together some training cycles that will get you started on the journey towards your first big total of the year. It's nice to have everything accounted for. Once the plan is in place, the only thing you have to do is find a way to improvise and adapt your plan when you encounter injuries… job changes… swine flu… unexpected pregnancies… gym closures… vehicle breakdowns… flash floods… earthquakes… family dramas… semester finals… Thanksgiving… and global terrorism. Maybe there are some things we can't plan for. Maybe we have to think on our feet and find quick ways to overcome disasters sometimes. Aye, there's the rub.

ALL GROWTH BEGINS WITH PAIN: PLANNING YOUR TRAINING, PART TWO

Last month's article took a broad look at competition planning. We examined some of the important issues a competitive weightlifter must address such as how many meets to compete in within a given year, anticipating distractions, and prioritizing which competitions are most important. That was step one. This month, we will be taking baby steps forward to the next step in the planning process.

Once a competition has been chosen and put on the calendar as one of your priorities for the year, it's time to plan out a training cycle that will produce the best possible results at the contest. For the sake of example, we will assume that the contest we are training for in this article is a national championship, top priority-type of situation. In other words, this is a meet where we want to hit the biggest lifts in our capability. This is not a training meet, and we will be specifically devoting a large time period to get ready for it. The qualifying total has already been made, the meet is a few months away, the travel arrangements have been figured out, the boss gave us the time off work, a neighbor has agreed to feed the dog while we're gone, and it's time to get in the gym and rock and roll. Now, once all of the general decisions have been made about how to approach this meet, the question that remains is how can we make sure that we are physically and mentally ready for a peak performance when the day of the contest arrives?

Training too hard in the early stages of the cycle will lead to peaking too early, and the contest will be a disaster. Not training hard enough will leave you soft and under-prepared on meet day, and the barbell will feel like you're hauling a 500 pound anchor off the bottom of the ocean when you pull it from the floor. Because you're a saucy little fireball and you've seen all the Rocky movies, your first inclination is simply to go to the gym and train absolutely as hard as you can every day. Push yourself to the maximum each time you put on your shoes, go to failure every day, try new personal records every week... I mean we're really going wild animal-style for this one, right?

You can train like that if you want to. Most likely, your body will feel great for a few weeks and then, most likely, you will run into a brick wall. Fatigue, injury, mental burnout and emotional destruction will leave you curled up in the fetal position and crying like a teenage girl whose mom just confiscated her Twilight books because you decided to train like a pack mule with no ideas about how to use patience and intelligence. Hey, don't feel bad if I just described your training life. I've been there and made every mistake I just listed, and then I ran into a coach who knew how to build champion weightlifters the way Jackson Pollack knew how to paint and get drunk.

Program design, friends. That's what we're talking about this month. Next month, we finish the trilogy with a look at how to structure a basic training week. And as always, we will provide information that will be beneficial to hardcore weightlifters and generalists alike.

First, the preamble...

Since 1992, I have been a member of the Calpian Weightlifting Club and coached by John Thrush. Because of this, much of the information I provide in these articles is heavily influenced by the "Calpian method." However, it is always important to mention that there are many weightlifting coaches out there and several of them have found different ways to effectively train athletes. I hate to use such a tired cliché, but there are many ways to skin a cat. This article would be just as credible if it was based on the methods of Gayle Hatch or Bob Takano. No coach has a monopoly on successful training methodology. But the Calpians have been one of the most accomplished weightlifting programs in America for twenty years and John Thrush is clearly one of the greatest coaches in the sport. That's why this information starts where it does. It is also crucial to state that the ideas in this article are not only from the Calpian approach. Several ideas from different coaches and programs will be used.

Now, down to business...

I'm a big fan of putting training plans down on paper. Most athletes like it when a coach gives them a typed program that tells them exactly how they will be training during the weeks leading up to a contest. Before the typing starts, let's get three important questions answered:

1) What weights does the athlete want to lift at the contest?
2) How many days a week will the athlete be able to train?
3) How many weeks are there until the contest?

We'll use a hypothetical lifter named Terry for this article, got it? The questions will be answered for Terry's particular abilities and circumstances.

1) What weights does Terry want to hit? Currently, Terry's best official competition lifts are 105 in the snatch and 140 in the clean and jerk.

At the contest we're training for, Terry expects to lift 110/145. His best back squat is 195 kilos and his best front squat is 170 kilos.

2) How many days a week will the athlete be able to train? Terry will train five days a week for this contest (Monday, Tuesday, Wednesday, Thursday, and Saturday)

3) How many weeks are there until the contest? There are twelve weeks.

One way to approach Terry's training is to set down a week-by-week loading schedule. This schedule tells us how much weight Terry will be lifting in training in the SN, C&J, rack jerks, squats, and pulls during the progressive weeks of the training cycle. For example, let's say we wanted to plan out the loading for his SN, C&J, and Back Squat. A graph for his loading schedule might look like this (sets and reps: 3x1 means three singles, 2x2 means two sets of two reps, 3x5 means three sets of five reps, etc.):

	SN	C&J	BSQ
Week 1	86 3x2	120 5x1	160 3x5
Week 2	88 3x2	122 5x1	165 2x5
Week 3	90 2x2	124 3x1	170 3x3
Week 4	93x2	126 3x1	174 3x3
Week 5	96x2	128 3x1	177 3x3
Week 6	85 3x1	115 3x1	181x3
Week 7	98x2	131 3x1	184x3
Week 8	100x2	134 2x1	188x2
Week 9	103x1	137x1	192x2
Week 10	106x1	140x1	195x2
Week 11	108x1	143x1	185 2x1
Week 12	Meet Week		

NOTES: These lifts are not all supposed to be performed on the same day, obviously. In next month's article, we will examine how to properly plan which exercises are trained on Monday, Tuesday, etc. This chart is set up to mean that sometime during week one, Terry has to snatch 86 kilos for three sets of two reps, C&J 120 for five singles, and back squat 160 for three sets of five.

Only the SN, C&J, and BSQ were planned in this example chart. For an actual program, the coach would want to plan out the loading progression for all the major exercises the lifter performs.

Only the top weights of the workout are listed on the chart. Warm-up sets are not included, but they are chosen at the athlete's discretion.

In the early weeks of the program, lighter weights are used with a higher number of repetitions. In the latter weeks, heavier weights are used with fewer repetitions.

The lightest weights at the beginning of the program are relatively light, but they are still above eighty percent of Terry's highest official lifts. When Terry sees this program, the first thought in his head will probably be that the 86 kilo snatches and 160 kilo squats in the early weeks are not heavy enough. The coach must instruct the athlete that this is a progressive overload program. Using progressive overload, the early weeks of the program deliberately include lighter weights because the athlete is building a foundation of speed and perfect technique through the use of multiple reps. As the weeks progress, the weights will gradually get heavier. This system should put Terry in a position to be stronger, fresher, and more technically sound than he has ever been when he gets to week twelve. The early weeks should also be a time when Terry successfully makes every attempt on his program, which is important in building the athlete's confidence. In other words, tell Terry that he's going to get plenty of shots at heavy weights in the coming weeks.

These weights are all educated guesses at what the athlete's capabilities will be on a given day. A wise coach will have some flexibility when it comes to watching the athlete and determining how much weight Terry should attempt in the workout. In other words, let's say we get to week nine and Terry is scheduled to snatch 103 on Monday. Terry is warming up and going through his workout, and he snatches 103 kilos like it's an empty bar. Terry is fired up, he feels good, and he wants to try 106 to break his personal record of 105. In that situation, my advice would be to put 106 on the bar and let Terry nail it. Even though he wasn't scheduled to snatch 106 until week ten, you have to strike while the iron is hot. If Terry misses the 106, the coach has to make a decision based on what the miss looked like. If Terry put a slow, dragging pull on the 106 and barely got it overhead before it came down and nearly decapitated him, I probably wouldn't advise more attempts at 106. I would tell Terry to go back down and snatch 96, then 101, and then possibly another shot at 106 if he is still looking sharp. The main point to remember is that you don't want to get trapped in the land where your athlete is missing snatch after snatch after snatch, and you're simply beating a dead horse. Sometimes, Terry might get lucky and nail the 106 after missing it eight times. More likely, he will continue missing and all the heavy attempts will leave him shot to hell for his next workout tomorrow.

Although it's important to be flexible, be smart in the early weeks of the program. If Terry is in week two and has just finished his fifth and last C&J single with 122, don't get carried away and say, "Jeez, that 122 was easy! Let's work up to 142!" Hold on, Jethro. The 122 was easy because it was supposed to be easy. Keep the leash on Terry for a few more weeks and let him strain against it like a dog who wants to run. When you finally cut the leash, he'll be primed and ready to explode.

For those of you who are not competitive weightlifters, this type of loading schedule is something you could use in your own workouts simply to get stronger and make progress. If you want to improve in any kind of measurable task, the theories and fundamentals of progressive overload training can make you better than you've ever been. If you're not an Olympic Lifter, but you like to bench press and you want to get stronger in it, then take the twelve-week cycle we just analyzed and use it for your bench training. You just might break through a barrier that's been holding you back.

Therefore...

All of this is designed to put Terry in a position where he will compete successfully and make 110/145 in the contest. If Terry makes all of the lifts on his program through week eleven, the coach might want to select his competition attempts as follows:

SN 1 - 103	C&J 1 - 137
SN 2 - 108	C&J 2 - 142
SN 3 - 110	C&J 3 - 145

Several variables could come into play here, obviously. If Terry is at the meet, he has just completed his second C&J with 142 and he has a chance to win the competition with 147, then it's time to deviate from the plan and put 147 on the bar. Likewise, let's say Terry's training hasn't gone well and he hasn't been able to snatch anything heavier than 100 prior to the meet. Given this situation, starting him with 103 would be a big roll of the dice. He might get lucky and hit the 103, but smart money would probably start him with a lighter weight that he has made consistently in training. Good coaches don't set up their athletes to bomb out.

What we can learn from all of this, and what we'll continue to learn next month in the third installment, is that good planning is good coaching. Knowing when to change the plan is also good coaching. And regardless of the fine points of your program or your particular area of strength training, the one overwhelming idea is that you simply have to be willing to work fiendishly hard if you want to get better. In Greek mythology, a man named Sisyphus was forced to spend eternity rolling a huge boulder up a hill. If he got lazy and relaxed, the boulder would roll down the hill and he would have to start all over again from the bottom. The idea here is that Sisyphus had to apply constant pressure and effort into pushing on the boulder. Any lapse in concentration or moment of weakness led to a setback. This is what training often feels like. This is what life often feels like. Building your business or raising your children becomes a constant battle where it feels like a gallon of effort only produces an inch of progress. It's difficult, challenging, and sometimes frustrating.

But if you want to look on the bright side, there is always an alternative to all the stress. You can always quit. Just grab that bag of Doritos and head for the couch. It'll be much easier there, no doubt about it. The only problem is that you're going to turn eighty someday, and you'll look back on your life and realize that your biggest accomplishment was owning the entire collection of The Rockford Files. If you don't want to end up that way, get behind that boulder and start pushing, baby.

SEVEN DAYS OF HEAVEN: PLANNING YOUR TRAINING, PART THREE

This will be the third and final installment in our three-part series on planning out your training. Two months ago, we examined the challenges of selecting goals and picking out competitions for a given year of training. Last month, we looked at the week-by-week loading progression for a training cycle that would lead up to one of those competitions. This month, we will narrow the subject down just a little more and take a look at how to set up a basic week of training. Seven days, seven days... The possibilities are endless.

Before we get into the meat of the subject, let's face reality. This is part three of a series of articles. And I think we all know the possible disasters that can occur when you get to a "part three" scenario. The Godfather Part III was a lousy movie. Return of the Jedi was the third part of the Star Wars trilogy and look at it, for crying out loud. You had a bunch of muppets running around killing storm troopers with homemade spears. Awful stuff, truly. Therefore, the goal here is to build up to a flaming climax. We want to make sure that this grand finale doesn't follow the sad tradition of third-part flops. Everybody should walk away from this month's article feeling like they could sit down at their computer and design a training program that will lead to continual progress, consistent strength development, injury-free training and new personal records.

Setting up a weekly training program presents you with some interesting demands because, as with all other elements of training, it will depend on the particular situation of the individual you're working with. What we will attempt to do here is put forward a weekly training plan and also address some ways that it could possibly be adapted or retooled to meet the needs of different athletes. Before we actually take a look at this weekly plan, it benefits us to throw out a few general training ideas that need to be taken into consideration.

Exercise Sequencing

Exercise sequencing, how's that for fancy terminology? It's almost like we have Mike Tyson here with us, creating his own vocabulary as he describes how ludicrous it is for his opponents to think they can depenetrate his impregnable defense. Praise be to Allah.

Exercise sequencing simply describes the order of your exercises in a given workout. If one workout is going to contain four exercises, which ones should be performed first and which ones should go last? For example, let's say an athlete wants to do snatches, back squats, some abdominal/core exercises, and clean pulls in one workout. What order should they follow?

Rule #1 Generally, the exercises that are most dependent on speed should be performed first. The athlete will be freshest and "snappiest" at the beginning of the workout before fatigue has set in from other exercises. Towards the end of a workout, after strenuous work has taken place, the athlete's explosiveness will be somewhat diminished. Trying to perform speed exercises at this point will not be optimal. In the workout example we're discussing here, which of the four exercises is most dependent on speed? The answer is obviously snatches. This means that the snatches should be done first.

Rule #2 Exercises that are closely movement-related should be performed in sequence. This means that if an athlete is going to perform snatches at the beginning of a workout, the exercises that immediately follow the snatches should be the ones that are most similar to the snatches. In this workout example, which exercise is the most movement-related to the snatches? The answer is the clean pulls. Although the snatch and the clean are different exercises, the triple extension of the pulling movement is a common factor between the two. After the athlete has finished doing snatches, the pulling movement will be "warmed up," so to speak. Because of this, the clean pulls are a good choice following the snatches because the pulling from the snatches will transfer into the clean pulls. Also, going back to Rule #1, the clean pulls are probably the second highest speed exercise in the workout. The snatches will be the most dependent on speed, and the clean pulls are second in the ranking order.

Rule #3 All of the barbell exercises should be completed before moving on to supplemental work. Having said this, the squats should be done after the clean pulls. After the squats are finished, the bar can be put away and the athlete can perform auxiliary exercises such as core strengthening, plyometrics, grip training, etc. Personally, I like to finish each workout with hanging leg raises, two or three other core exercises such as crunches or planks, and crush gripper training. I also like to stretch for ten minutes after each workout. Post-workout stretching should be a permanent part of your training program. Therefore, the workout should look like this:

1) Snatch
2) Clean Pulls

3) Squats
4) Core/Abdominal work
5) Stretching

Variations

These rules are effective guides for planning your workouts. However, it must always be stated that adding some occasional variety and changing things up can pay big dividends. For example, I once decided that I was going to experiment with performing my strength work at the beginning of my workouts, followed by my speed lifts. I deliberately wanted to be fatigued from heavy strength lifts (squats) prior to the speed exercises such as snatches or clean and jerks. The idea here was that when I finally got to a competition and performed snatches and clean and jerks without the pre-fatigue from squats, my explosiveness would be greater. In other words, the bar would feel lighter on meet day. I trained like this for around six weeks and then went to a meet. Did it work? I don't think I noticed a big physical change, either positive or negative. I basically felt the same on meet day as I usually had in other meets. But it was fun to train differently for a while. I once snatched 140 kilos (around 90% of my max) immediately after back squatting 250x5, and I think there was a mental benefit from this because I basically started believing that I could snatch 90% anytime, anywhere, regardless of anything.

OFF DAYS!!!

You might decide that you want to train seven days a week. I wouldn't, but you can if you want to. If you choose to go this route, you won't need to worry about off days because you won't have any (until you enter the hospital).

But for those of you who are trying to decide how many days a week to train and which days you should take off, here are a few thoughts. First of all, you have to ask the question, "How many days a week should I train?" If you talk to ten different coaches about this, you'll probably get ten different answers. I've known elite lifters who train six days a week, and I've known elite lifters who train three days a week. There is no rule set in stone that applies to everybody. When I was doing the best lifting of my career, I trained five days a week. After a few years of this, I changed to four days a week and guess what? I continued to do the best lifting of my career and even made some solid improvements.

As we have said repeatedly in our series, things are dependent on your personal schedule. Your job might completely dictate how many days a week you can train. If you have a job that only allows you to get to the gym three days a week, then you will have to set up a three-day-per-week program. Nothing complicated there. But if you're in the fortunate position of having as much time as you need to train, then the questions really begin. Selecting which days are going to be your off days is a strategic move. Logically, it makes sense that you will want to take your off days when you will need them the most. How can we accurately gauge when that will be?

Sundays

I've taken Sundays off throughout my entire career, and I think most lifters do as well. Some people have religious obligations that prohibit them from training on Sundays. Some people believe that weightlifting is their religion. Regardless, Sunday is generally a good off day because it freshens up the athlete for the coming week. There's a sense of completion that accompanies Sundays. A feeling tends to come over people that tells them their work for the week is done and it's time to relax, mentally unwind, and enjoy the day before the grind starts again on Monday. This is probably why NFL games are televised on Sundays. They practically force America to the couch. One of the best lifters I've ever trained with told me, "If you're a lifter, Sundays are for laying down, eating, and napping." Truer words have never been spoken.

Between D-Day and Armageddon

There should always be a day off between two workouts that are extremely demanding. One way of approaching this is to arrange your most difficult workouts around an off day. For example, you could plan an off day on a Wednesday if you know that you're really going to be hitting it hard on Tuesday and Thursday. If you're planning to take Sundays off, as we mentioned earlier, then it makes sense that Saturday and Monday would be big workouts. The overall thought here is that there has to be a structure to your training week. Off days should not be random. If you have a job situation where you know that you won't be able to train on Saturdays and Sundays, then your Friday and Monday workouts should be the ones where you plan to get the most intense work accomplished.

Finally, an example...

Now, with all those theories and rules lying on the table, let's just quit beating around the bush and put one week of training down on paper. Here it is:

Monday
- Cleans
- Clean Pulls
- Back Squats
- Straight-Legged Deadlifts
- Abs

Tuesday
- Rack Jerks
- Power Cleans
- Standing Military Press
- Abs

Wednesday
- Snatches
- Snatch Pulls
- Abs

Thursday
- Clean and Jerks
- Clean Pulls
- Stop Squats
- Straight-Legged Deadlifts
- Abs

Saturday
- Snatches
- Snatch Pulls
- Front Squats
- Abs

I didn't list stretching in any of these workouts, but it should be included in all of them.

There you go. Now, let's take a look at some reasons for why this week looks the way it does.

Thursday and Saturday are big workouts, hence the day off on Friday. Plus, the athlete will be training four days in a row throughout the week (Mon-Thurs), so he/she will be ready for a day off by Friday. Sunday is a day off for the reasons already mentioned.

Three squat workouts per week is a good plan for a competitive Olympic lifter. Some coaches actually have their athletes squat four or five times per week, with more moderate weights. I personally have found that doing three squat workouts per week and really hitting those workouts hard will be most effective.

Doing rack jerks on a day that follows a squat workout is part of the design. The legs will be fatigued the day after squats. Performing rack jerks when the legs are fatigued simulates how the athlete will feel during a heavy competition clean and jerk, where the legs will be fatigued after standing up with the heavy clean. If the athlete can adapt and learn to use the legs in the jerk effectively on Tuesday after the tough Monday squat workout, there will be a benefit in the full clean and jerk.

Following the competition lifts with a pulling exercise is a good way to strengthen the movement. In other words, always do clean pulls after cleans. Always do snatch pulls after snatches, etc.

Straight-Legged Deadlifts are designed to strengthen the lower back, stretch the hamstrings, and prevent injury. This exercise does not need to be performed with enormous weights. It is performed with a barbell, but it should be viewed as an auxiliary exercise.

Adaptations

This program is specifically designed for athletes who are completely concentrating on Olympic Weightlifting. If the athlete is planning to incorporate other athletic endeavors into their training, such as running or mountain biking, then the program would need to be restructured. The intensity and workload of this program will not leave much energy left for additional pursuits.

Age issues must be considered. I would not have a thirty year-old athlete train five days a week in this manner. If a thirty year-old wanted to train five days a week, the intensity of the workouts would need to be reduced. I've trained at twenty years old and I've trained at thirty years old. The simple fact is that the body just doesn't recover as quickly as the years pass by.

In this particular training week, the two competition lifts (snatch/clean and jerk) are not trained on the same day. This is simply a basic look at how to build a training week. For a competitive weightlifter, it is important to train the competition lifts together on the same day to simulate actual meet conditions. This training week would need to be organized a bit differently to accommodate that principle.

There are a few other things I would like to add about this program, along with program design in general. First of all, the five-day training week I outlined in this article looks very simple. There aren't any magic exercises in there. In fact, some people might take a look at it and think that it doesn't look like enough work to make big progress. I've shown this training week to several lifters over the years and had them give me the same response, "Wow, this doesn't look very hard."

Okay... When I moved to Washington in 1993 to train with the Calpian Weightlifting Club, I began using the exact same five-day plan I described in this article. It was very different from how I had trained in the past, but I had been stuck at the same weights for over a year and I needed a change. I came to Washington in January and had a best competition total of 265 kilos in the 99 kilo class. After eleven months of training this way every week, I totaled 300 kilos at the same bodyweight. Now, it's important to understand that I was pushing myself extremely hard within this framework, as were all the lifters in our club. Our coach had our daily workout weights planned out throughout our entire program, but we were not hesitant about deviating from the plan and loading up personal records on the bar if the time was right to go for it (remember last month's article?). It was a sensible, organized approach that also encouraged aggressiveness and breaking new ground. All of the information from this article, along with the preceding two articles in this series, give you a solid idea of how I've trained throughout my career and how I've trained other athletes.

And because of our thousand-ways-to-skin-a-cat understanding, it's important to acknowledge that this isn't the only way to train successfully. Can you go from 265 to 300 in one year training differently than how I've discussed? Absolutely. Weightlifting coaches sometimes make the same mistake as some religious leaders: they basically say, "Only I am right, everyone else is wrong." The point that I hope we all understand is that there are certain commonalities that make for smart training, even if the daily routines are dissimilar. Despite individual differences in workout frequency, loading progression and exercise selection, every coach will have to use some good old-fashioned horse sense when it comes to program design. "Horse sense," for those of you who weren't lucky enough to grow up in the boondocks, is a term that refers to sound practical judgment. Sound practical judgment, along with a fantastic work ethic, unrelenting commitment, and high pain tolerance will usually make you a better athlete, coach, spouse, parent, professional, or Jedi Knight. So file down your calluses and get to work, and may the force be with you.

SNATCH PULLS AND THE LOCH NESS MONSTER: A LOOK AT SOME OF THE FACT AND FICTION OF WEIGHTLIFTING

My grandfather tells me that Adolph Hitler is still alive. In fact, my grandfather knows exactly where he lives. One of the men I work with tells me that George Bush personally planned the 9/11 attacks, all the way down to the hiring of the terrorists who hijacked the planes. A weightlifter I used to train with once told me that my elbows would feel better if I found a way to hook them up to a car battery between workouts. One of my uncles once told me that you should never marry somebody who is better looking than you are.

I believe one of those statements is true, and I think the rest of them are all pig vomit. But the longer you live and the more people you meet in the world, the more pieces of information you'll hear. Some of them will make a lot of sense and you'll believe them right away. Others will sound so stupid that you immediately classify them as false. And then there are the occasional tidbits that you're not entirely sure about. They definitely sound a little shaky, but there is enough sense in them to give you pause and stick an ongoing question into your brain.

Weightlifting is, without a doubt, a sport where you will hear a lot of these tidbits. First of all, you have to know that almost everybody you meet in weightlifting will consider himself an expert on it. The ones with more years and experience in the sport will often think that only they are right and everyone who disagrees with them is retarded. In any case, you will never, ever have trouble finding a weightlifter who isn't willing to tell you everything you need to know about training, competing, how to fix US Weightlifting, how to beat the Chinese, how to file your taxes, how to keep from losing your hair, how to win the Super Bowl, etc. Our sport is the mothership of mental giants who can fix your life if you'll just listen to them and learn.

Knowing this, we can use this article to throw out a few popular weightlifting ideas and classify them as fact or fiction. I am absolutely not going to try to convince any of you that I have all the answers on everything. I'll even go a step further and admit that there are a few areas where I'm as clueless as a sorority girl at a Mensa convention. Being handsome is a mystery to me, for example. Hell, I was just born that way. I don't know how it happens. However, being a weightlifter for many years has given me the chance to know a thing or two about a thing or two. So here we go...

Fact Vs. Fiction

Statement Bulgarian weightlifters don't use pulls as part of their training. Fact or fiction?

Fiction Some of the Bulgarian lifters use pulls in their training. There has been a common conception about the Bulgarian method over the years: Most people believe that their approach is completely stripped down to using the snatch, clean and jerk, and front squat in training. No assistance exercises, almost no back squats, no pulls, etc. This is what you frequently hear when you read weightlifting forums on the internet. One of the reasons people think this is true is that there are several training hall videos of the Bulgarians available through Randall Strossen's IronMind company and, in most of those videos, you only see the Bulgarians performing the competition lifts, the front squat, and the back squat. Right away, that dispels the front-squat-only myth about them. Every Bulgarian training video I have ever seen, and I've seen most of them, shows a lot of back squatting. And in regards to the no-pulls myth, Strossen has a Bulgarian training video available on IronMind that shows Zlatan Vanev doing snatch pulls in the training hall of the 1996 Olympics. Apparently, they do use pulls in their training. It might very well be true that the Bulgarians don't use pulls with much frequency. But many lifting enthusiasts take this idea and run with it, eliminating pulls from their training because "that's how the Bulgarians do it, and the Bulgarians are the best!" Because it's in my nature to be "skeptical up the receptacle" as Don King once said, I'll suggest that the Bulgarians probably do a lot of things that aren't necessarily a good idea for every weightlifter. I certainly wouldn't take their advice on how to pass a drug test, for example. Their methods have produced some of the most phenomenal results in the history of our sport. There is no denying that. But there is also no denying the fact that the Bulgarians have a dark side to their training that has led to some of the most shameful controversies in the history of our sport. I think it's important to look at all the angles when thinking about how to train. Bulgarian weightlifting has more angles than an architectural textbook.

Statement It's better to lift without the use of any supportive equipment (wrist wraps, belts, knee sleeves). Fact or fiction?

Fact But this one has an asterisk next to it. Most lifters begin their training, or *should* begin their training, wearing only their workout clothes and a pair of weightlifting shoes. If the lifter continues to train and time goes by and the lifter never feels any soreness in the wrists, back or knees, then there is no need to add any equipment. Now, this is the real world and it has to be acknowledged that there will be times in many weightlifters' careers when they develop this soreness and stiffness in these areas; when these pains surface, using wrist wraps, Rehband knee sleeves, or a weightlifting belt can allow the lifter to continue to train. There is nothing wrong with this. At different times in my career, I have used all of these pieces of equipment. There were times when my wrists were so sore that I don't think I could have made it through the workouts without wrist wraps. However, lifters should also be willing to get rid of equipment when they don't need it anymore. After a few years, I decided to stop using wrist wraps and my wrists were fine without them. I also used to wear knee sleeves, and then I eventually stopped using them. Now, I'm thirty-six and the only equipment I use is a belt when I do heavy squats or clean and jerks. I don't wear anything when I snatch. Interestingly, my body actually feels better now than it did back when I was using more equipment. The image that pops into my head is watching Ronny Weller compete at the 2000 Olympics. For those of you who don't know, Weller is one of the legendary lifters of our sport and his list of major injuries throughout his career would make you cringe. But there he stood in 2000, at thirty-one years of age, snatching 210 and totaling 467.5 wearing nothing but his lifting suit, a t-shirt, and his shoes. He found a way to train without equipment. Now, he was beaten at that Olympics by Hossein Rezazedeh, who was wearing a belt, wrist wraps, and knee wraps. Which method is the correct one? Neither. One lifter needed to use equipment and the other one didn't. If you don't need it, don't wear it. If you need it, wear it. Just don't be afraid to get rid of it if you find that you can.

Statement Upper body pressing strength is important for jerking successfully. Fact or fiction?

Fiction The jerk is dependent on the strength and power of the lower body, not the deltoids, triceps, etc. Using the muscles of the legs, hips, and core to drive the bar off the shoulders is the secret to jerking. In fact, many elite lifters do not have phenomenal pressing strength because they don't use presses in training. Overhead pressing can be a useful supplemental exercise and having a strong upper body is certainly going to be a benefit to any strength athlete. (Let's never forget what we're doing here. We're lifting weights. Being strong is a good thing.) However, relying on the muscles of the upper body to elevate the bar in the jerk is a recipe for failure. I once had a conversation with Wes Barnett about pressing strength. Wes had a best official clean and jerk of 220 kilos and my best was 185. I used military presses (strict form) in training occasionally and I mentioned that the top press I could do was 105 kilos. Interestingly, Wes told me that his top press was probably around the same weight. 105 kilos/231 pounds is not impressive pressing strength when you consider that many elite bench pressers can do strict military presses with over 300 pounds. But I was able to jerk over 400 pounds and Wes could do close to 500 pounds because of technique, speed, and power from the lower body.

Statement Many of the top lifters in the world squat with lighter weights than the massive poundages you hear rumors about. Fact or fiction?

Fact Most of the rumors you hear about the squatting numbers of the best lifters in the world are greatly exaggerated. When I began weightlifting, I was told by one of the top US lifters of the time that Soviet world champion Alexander Kurlovich could front squat 400 kilos for two reps. This was a lifter who had been on some international trips to Europe and rubbed elbows with the world champions, so he definitely seemed like a knowledgeable source. Years later, I read an interview with Kurlovich himself where he stated that his top back squat was 350 kilos. Now, 350 kilos is 771 pounds. By any standard, this is a jaw-dropping amount of weight, especially when you consider the strict form and depth used by the world's top Olympic Lifters. However, a 350 kilo back squat is much different from the 400x2 front squat that I originally heard about of Kurlovich. This same exaggeration exposure has happened with Leonid Taranenko and Anatoly Pisarenko when they candidly reported their top back squats. These men don't circulate misinformation. Misinformation gets circulated by others on their behalf. Pisarenko, interestingly, has one of the highest clean and jerks in history (265 kilos) and he has personally stated that he rarely squatted with heavier weights than he could clean and jerk. This is not to say that leg strength is unimportant, obviously. Leg strength is one of the most critical factors in weightlifting success. Any expert would agree to that. However, the common notion among the weightlifting crowd is that the top Olympic Lifters in the world can regularly squat weights that are in excess of the squat world records from powerlifting. This is not true. If you travel to Russia and visit a national training center, you will see some insanely strong weightlifters who have some of the most powerful legs in the world. But many Americans believe that those Russian lifters are loading the bar up to 900 pounds on a daily basis and knocking out sets of three like they're doing deep knee bends with a broomstick. This is simply not true.

And there's more where that came from...

This article would be longer than *Gone With the Wind* if we threw every weightlifting rumor we've ever heard on the table. Even if you're a relative newbie in the sport, you've most likely come across some pretty substantial eyebrow-raisers. The tricky thing about these little chunks of information is that all of them have a devoted faithful following. Every misconception is gospel truth to somebody. Try convincing my grandpa that Hitler is dead. See where that gets you. Or better yet, try approaching some of the old-timers you meet at weightlifting meets and tell them that upper body strength is not crucial to weightlifting success. These are the senior members of our crowd who used to watch ABC Wide World of Sports when Serge Reding and Vasily Alexeev were pressing (if you want to call what they did back then "presses") over 500 pounds and dagnabit, those guys were the REAL weightlifters, sonny! Even as this article comes to a close, I'm positive that somebody who reads it is going to seriously disagree with one of the claims I've made. And it's fine if we disagree. Because unlike many of my weightlifting brethren, I'm not the definitive expert on every subject under the sun. I mean really... I married a woman who is much better looking than me. What do I know about anything?

PRAYING

I was coaching at the Junior National Weightlifting Championships back in the 90s; can't remember the exact year. In one session, there was a young guy who was attempting a clean and jerk that would have earned him a bronze medal if he made it. He had already attempted the lift twice and failed both times because of press-out. These were horrible press-outs, too. Very strong kid but absolutely terrible jerk technique. On his last attempt, he cleaned the weight, jerked it with the biggest press-out I've ever seen, and then put the weight down and started to walk off the platform. He must have thought he was going to get credit for the lift, because he was stood there looking at the scoreboard where the red and white lights flash after the lift is completed. White lights mean the judges say the lift is good, red lights mean you did something wrong and the lift is no good. As this kid waited for the lights to flash, he was loudly yelling, "PLEASE GOD! PLEASE GOD! PLEASE GOD!" Then the lights came up red (meaning the lift was no good) and he screamed out, "GOD DAMN IT!!!!" I think it might have been the only time in my life where I saw somebody go from asking god for something to completely rejecting their religious beliefs in a space of three seconds.

TWO ROADS DIVERGED: A LOOK AT THE CONVERSION FROM POWERLIFTING TO WEIGHTLIFTING

Powerlifters and Olympic Weightlifters love to engage in verbal brawls. These brawls are almost always centered on the question of "Who is *really* stronger… powerlifters or weightlifters?" No matter how many voices of reason attempt to intervene with the idea that the two sports are simply quite different and difficult to compare, most coaches and athletes in both sports will throw rational thinking out the window and dive into a conversation that closely resembles two cavemen clubbing each other in the head with dinosaur bones. These exchanges pop up in articles and internet message boards quite often. But despite the fact that these arguments are frequent, it is noticeably rare to see athletes from powerlifting or weightlifting actually attempt to cross the great divide and convert from one sport to the other. Most powerlifters never try weightlifting, and most weightlifters never try powerlifting.

However, there have been some amazing examples of crossover success. The two most popular case studies in this department, and the favorite arguments of the powerlifting faithful, are the accomplishments of Mark Henry and Shane Hamman. Both Mark and Shane were record-holders in powerlifting with some behemoth numbers to their credit. They both left their squat/bench/deadlift days behind and became Olympic Weightlifters, and they both won multiple national championships on the way to becoming Olympians. So, does this mean that every strength athlete who attempts to convert to a different sport will have the same success as Mark and Shane? The answer is clearly "NO" because not every athlete has it in their destiny to make an Olympic Team. But the question remains, "If lifters decide to convert from one sport to another, can they expect to have success?" The answer is a complicated one with several variables to consider. This article will examine my own personal experience in this area along with some analysis of the basic challenges associated with jumping the strength sport fence.

The Reasons for Converting

Why would an athlete want to walk away from a sport they have trained seriously and competed in, especially if the athlete is talented and has tasted success? Furthermore, why would an athlete leave a familiar sport to move into a new area where he/she has to go back to being a newbie and start from the bottom again? Each individual has their own reasons and they are all unique, but my personal journey from powerlifting to weightlifting began with some internal conflicts about what I wanted to accomplish as an athlete. First, a little background information is needed. I began competing in powerlifting when I was fifteen years old and, fortunately, I experienced quick success. Less than a year after my first competition, I won the high school national championship and broke several state records in my age division. I continued competing and training for two years and I was able to make significant progress with no real coaching or training partners. However, there were certain elements of powerlifting that I could not get comfortable with. These issues become the foundation for my move to Olympic Weightlifting.

First, I was bothered by the supportive gear used in powerlifting. I competed in the late 1980s, long before the use of support gear was the complex science it has become today. But even back in those days, lifters were using squat suits and bench shirts to add huge numbers to their competition lifts. I used this gear myself. And even though I wore my suits/shirt loosely, I still knew that there was absolutely no way that I would be able to squat or bench the same weights if I was wearing shorts and a t-shirt. For whatever reason, this bothered me extensively and I considered it a shot to my pride. The second major issue in powerlifting that I could not swallow was the existence of multiple federations in the sport that all conducted their own state, national, and world championships. In my opinion, this situation cheapened the title of "National Champion" or "World Champion." If there were six or seven other lifters in my weight class who had also won national championships in different federations, how could any of us legitimately state that we were the best in the United States? At one point, my deadlift was an official national record in my age division and bodyweight class. But I knew that there were other federations where athletes of my same age and weight had deadlifted more than me, so the record was a hollow one. All of these factors might not have been bothersome to most athletes, but they certainly did not sit well with me.

However, I gradually began learning and reading more about the sport of Olympic Weightlifting during my powerlifting years. All of the problems of supportive gear and multiple federations did not exist in weightlifting. There was one state champion, one national champion, one world champion, and these champions won their titles with their muscles and talent instead of using the newest triple-ply bench shirt that added thirty extra pounds to their competition total. In my perspective, the sport was a much more pure test of skill and a much more definitive test of who the best lifters really were. And as an additional piece of bait, the chance to compete in the Olympics someday was a magical thought. The Olympic Games are the most sacred sports event in the history of the planet, and powerlifting is not a part of it.

Therefore, the allure was there. The excitement and interest in trying to conquer a new area was in place. Still, the obvious question remained, "What does it take to convert from powerlifting to weightlifting?"

Mental and Physical Obstacles

When I decided to try Olympic Weightlifting, it almost seemed like it was going to be too easy. This idea started when I picked up a copy of IronMan Magazine in 1988 and read an article about how a weightlifter named Dean Goad had recently done a 365 pound clean and jerk in the 165 pound class, and that lift was a new junior national record. "365 pounds?" I thought. "I can deadlift over 500. I know it's tougher to put the bar over your head, like in the clean and jerk. But I'll bet I can do 365 because deadlifting 500 is easy!"

It is not difficult to see where this story is leading. The first time I attempted to do an Olympic Lift, it was all very simple. I went to the gym, put 135 pounds on the bar, tried to clean it, and fell over backwards with the bar landing on my femur. All of a sudden, that old bench shirt seemed very, very comfortable.

There are several obstacles involved in transitioning over from powerlifting to Olympic Lifting. One of the biggest and most important obstacles is simply *finding a coach*. Because of the relative simplicity of the powerlifting movements, I had been able to make fast progress in the sport without having a coach's eyes on me. Many successful powerlifters do not even use coaches. Weightlifting, on the other hand, is extremely complex and incredibly difficult to learn if there is no coach present to teach the basics of the snatch and clean and jerk. And even if a powerlifter is able to find a good coach to teach the Olympic movements, the mental battle is a fierce one. Going from being an athlete who can easily hit a 500 pound squat to being an athlete who is getting owned by a 150 pound snatch is humbling, to say the least. If the athlete is hungry and competitive, as most strength athletes are, the process can be maddening. The athlete has to have patience to learn the Olympic lifts. If the athlete has no patience, it will be force-fed during the learning process.

And then, if the athlete is persistent enough to find a competent coach, the physical challenges begin to surface. For most former powerlifters, flexibility is a problem. The usual culprit areas are the wrists, elbows, shoulders, hip flexors, and ankles. Because of the relatively short range of motion in the power lifts, the muscles and connective tissue often develop in a way that creates stiffness and, in some cases, prohibitive or "muscle-bound" lack of flexibility. The longer the athlete has spent intensely training the bench press and powerlifting-style squats, the more limited the flexibility is likely to be. I had two factors that benefited me when I converted: a) I was only 18 and had not lost my ankle flexibility yet and b) I was not heavily muscled in the upper body. This second factor worked against me as a powerlifter because I was a weak bench presser. But in weightlifting, it was a positive attribute because I had solid lock-out in the elbows and I was able to fix the bar comfortably over my ears when performing snatches or jerks. Any powerlifter who has a severe lack of flexibility prior to beginning weightlifting training will have to begin with an extensive stretching program. All of the stretching that is performed in this program should be directed towards attaining the positions of the snatch and clean and jerk. Generally speaking, pre-workout stretching should be more ballistic and post-workout stretching should be more static. The positives and negatives of both types of stretching are outlined in Greg Everett's *Olympic Weightlifting: A Complete Guide for Athletes & Coaches*. It is worth mentioning that I did a large amount of intense pre-workout static stretching in my early career, and I suffered frequent muscle pulls and partial tears during training. These injuries became much less frequent when I abandoned pre-workout static stretching and moved to more ballistic, movement-centered stretching.

Interestingly, the conversion process from powerlifting to weightlifting is when it becomes obvious that there are different *types* of strength involved in both sports. Here is an example. When I was a powerlifter, my strongest lift was the deadlift. It is clear that the pulling movement of the deadlift relies heavily on the back muscles. Because of this, I concluded that I had a strong back. However, when I began training the Olympic lifts, I had an extremely difficult time keeping my back flat and tight. Heavy cleans and front squats would put me in the "turtle-back" position where the spine is rounded and the elbows are collapsing forward. It made no sense to me because the turtle-back problem indicated that I had a lack of back strength, along with a weak overall core. How could I have a lack of back strength if I had an outstanding deadlift?

The answer is that a strong back in powerlifting does not necessarily guarantee proper positions in the Olympic lifts. The muscles of the spinal erectors, trapezius, latissimus, and infraspinatus have to be developed in a very particular way to keep the strict, flat-back position necessary for the Olympic lifts. These muscles are not going to be developed in the correct manner if they have been trained to haul up maximum deadlifts in a grinding, rounded-back fashion. The only way the transition can be made is through extended training where the athlete pays constant attention to detail and physically forces him/herself to maintain a flat back posture. After hundreds and hundreds of reps with light weights where the muscles are required to contract in a way that keeps the back as flat as a board, the athlete will eventually be able to maintain proper positions.

The Process of Training and Competing

To make the transition even more complicated, the issue of developing an effective training program must be tackled. It is worth mentioning that this was a much bigger problem around 1990 than it is now because of the internet. These days, a new lifter can Google "Olympic Weightlifting" and come up with a variety of sample training programs and message boards where there will be mountains of information. Twenty years ago, it was much more difficult. I can recall having to mail (no, not e-mail… MAIL) coaches around the state and ask for help with training programs.

Fortunately, there were a few good coaches who were willing to show me the bare bones of a training program involving sets and reps, pulling exercises, volume/intensity in the squats, etc. The routine I used in the early days was not terribly complex:

Monday	Tuesday	Wednesday	Thursday	Saturday
Snatch	Rack Jerks	Cleans	Snatch	CJ
Clean Pulls	Power Cleans	Snatch Pulls	Clean Pulls	Snatch Pulls
Stop Squats	Pressing	Abs	Front Squats	Back Squats
Abs	Abs		Abs	Abs

This was the general outline I used. I almost always did doubles and singles in the competition lifts and triples in the pulls/squats. However, the weights I used on a daily basis were problematic because my approach was very simple; I went as heavy as I possibly could in every exercise every day, often not stopping until I had missed several attempts or had a mental meltdown, or both. I still had no coach to work with me for the first two years and the idea of using light weights to improve my technique seemed morally wrong (remember, I was eighteen years old and on my own). Needless to say, minor injuries and failed attempts quickly became a consistent part of my training. It would have been extremely helpful to hold back on the weights in the early days and focus entirely on positions as opposed to poundage. Looking back now, I should have spent a great deal of time practicing snatches and clean and jerks with an empty bar or PVC pipe in the beginning.

Also, one of the notable problems from those days is that I spent a lot of time working on power snatches and power cleans instead of forcing myself to perform the full movements. I believed that power snatches and cleans would make me better at finishing the pull. And, of course, I was much more likely to miss a lift if I tried to perform the full version because of my inexperience and rough technique in the bottom position. As with many beginners, I could power snatch more than I could full snatch. With these two considerations, I probably performed 70-80% of all my training lifts as power movements. The obvious result is that I was very good at power snatches and power cleans, but I had shown little improvement in the full lifts. My idea that performing power movements would make me better at finishing the pull was partially correct, I believe. But the pull is obviously only part of the movement. The receiving position of a full lift has to be trained and memorized by the motor system as precisely as the pull does.

However, even with all these early mistakes, there are still a few positive ideas from the transition process that I would recommend to potential converts. One of these ideas is jump training. I did quite a bit of plyometric work during my first two years of training the Olympic lifts because all of the literature I read indicated that Olympic Weightlifters had tremendous jumping ability. I would usually finish each workout with a few sets of box jumps and depth jumps to improve explosiveness. As with anything else, it is entirely possible to do too much jump training and I definitely did too much. Patellar tendonitis was not far behind. However, the basic idea of using jump training in the early part of an Olympic lifting program is essential, especially if the athlete has a prior background in a sport that emphasizes slow movements like powerlifting. It simply has to be incorporated into the training program with some planning and common sense.

In addition to all of these training considerations, the questions of competition should be addressed. When is an athlete ready to compete, and how frequently should he/she compete in the early stages of training? Different coaches will obviously have different philosophies on this. My personal idea is that athletes should begin competing as soon as they have a strong command of the movements. When they can perform snatches and clean and jerks with a solid level of technical proficiency, let them enter meets and compete. However, beginners should have their attempts chosen very carefully. The competition goals of beginners should be A) go six-for-six and B) set new personal records. Winning trophies and medals should be emphasized less than personal performance, because most newcomers will likely be beaten by more experienced lifters in their early meets. Additionally, it is the coach's job to instruct the athlete on *how to compete*. No athlete should shy away from tough competition. If a rookie enters a first meet and happens to be competing against an experienced national level lifter, the rookie will be demoralized if the coach has emphasized winning as the primary goal. At my first competition, I competed against a national champion who beat me by 115 kilos. Instead of being discouraged, I was inspired by the huge weights I had seen this athlete lift. I walked away from the meet saying to myself, "I want to be as good as that guy some day." Newbies should be energized by seeing incredible performances, and it is the coach's job to teach that idea. I also believe that newcomers should compete frequently. It is essential that the athlete gains experience and develops a sense of being in control on the competition platform. This will happen if the athlete gets a lot of "platform time" and completes a lot of successful lifts.

Overall Perspective

After the swelling has been iced and the chalk has settled, the question remains; "If lifters decide to convert from one sport to another, can they expect to have success?" The answer is that *it all depends on the athlete*. As mentioned, there are a variety of physical variables that have to be examined such as flexibility, elbow lockout, coordination, agility, and others. Long-term powerlifting training can certainly put the athlete behind the eight ball when it comes time to convert to Olympic Weightlifting because these physical variables are developed so much differently than they need to be for Olympic success. Physically, there are some athletes that are clearly "naturals." Mark Henry snatched 150 kilos in the first weightlifting meet he competed in. That is a fairly strong indicator of physical potential.

However, as any weightlifter can tell you, having the body is only half the battle. You also have to have the brain. After twenty years of competing, training, and coaching, I now subscribe to the idea that there are two types of talent: physical and mental. And no athlete can be successful without a long supply of both. Weightlifting will not forgive laziness or lack of discipline. Unfortunately, it will also not forgive a lack of athletic ability. The sport will strenuously test every physical and personality trait you possess. It is the individual journey of the athlete to make a complete commitment, press the gas pedal to the floor, and see how far the journey goes.

PULLING, PUSHING, AND THINKING: EXTENDED CONNECTIONS BETWEEN OLYMPIC LIFTING AND POWERLIFTING

My earliest workout routines are very clear in my memory. I started lifting weights at the high school weight room when I was thirteen with some of the kids I played football with. We developed our own training program, based on some advanced scientific principles and theories. Here is a rough skeleton of our normal training week:

Monday	Tuesday	Wednesday	Thursday	Friday
Bench Press	Bench Press	Bench Press	Bench Press	Bench Press
Curls	Curls	Curls	Curls	Curls
Wrestle	Go home	Hit each other	Wrestle	Shoplift

For better or for worse, thousands of young athletes in this country become enthusiastic about weight training because they are obsessed with the bench press. If the athletes are young and have no guidance from any coaches (which we didn't), it is an easy trap to fall into. However, I was lucky enough to learn squatting and deadlifting shortly after I started working out. It didn't take long for these lifts to replace my obsession with bench pressing. I did not learn the Olympic Lifts until the summer after my high school graduation.

This article will revisit the subject of connecting the power lifts (squat, bench press, deadlift) with the Olympic lifts (snatch, clean and jerk). There are millions of athletes who use a combination of these two disciplines to gain strength and overall athleticism. Likewise, there are millions of athletes who completely specialize in powerlifting or Olympic Weightlifting for competitive purposes. Converting from one sport to another has already been examined in a previous *Performance Menu* issue. However, there are many other nuggets of information lying in the dirt. My own personal experience and the experiences of other athletes will dust these nuggets off and give us a better look at them.

Pull for your freedom!

One of the simplest commonalities between Olympic lifting and powerlifting is the pull from the floor. The technique used in deadlifting and cleaning/snatching has several similarities and, admittedly, several differences. However, every athlete wants to improve their pulling strength regardless of the particular movement. Here is where we find an interesting truth; training the pull as an Olympic lifter can dramatically improve the powerlifting deadlift.

There are two personal examples that will better illustrate this idea. When I was seventeen, I had trained the deadlift specifically for four years. I had never done any Olympic movements. At this time, my best deadlift was an absolute gut-busting 535 pounds. Then, after I graduated high school, a coach taught me the Olympic lifts and how to train as a full-time Olympic lifter. I was hooked, so I completely abandoned powerlifting and concentrated on Olympic lifting. My training program was very basic. I practiced the competition lifts every day, did front/back squats, and did clean/snatch pulls three times every week. The heaviest pulling I ever did was around 150 kilos (330 pounds) in the clean pulls and 120 kilos (264 pounds) in the snatch pulls. And these weights were the absolute heaviest I would ever pull; my pulling weights were often lighter than these. My top squat workout weights during this time were usually around 400-420 pounds.

I had trained this way for ten months. I had not done a single deadlift during this time. Then one day I decided to do some deadlifts, just for the hell of it. I deadlifted 555 pounds easily that day, which was a 20 pound improvement over my old personal best from when I was focusing on the deadlift. I simply could not believe that my pulling strength had increased so much because I had not been pulling heavy weights for almost a full year. However, that was not the only time I saw this happen in my career.

After the day when I deadlifted 555 pounds, I went back to full-time Olympic lifting and did not deadlift again for ten years. During this decade, my Olympic lifting career moved forward steadily as I fought to climb up in the national rankings. I eventually achieved a 155 kilo snatch and a 185 kilo clean and jerk. My top back squat during this time was 245 kilos (540 pounds), and I continued to utilize clean/snatch pulls three times per week in training. The heaviest weights I ever used in the clean pulls were around 205 kilos (451 pounds) and around 165 kilos (363 pounds) in the snatch pulls. And again, my weights in these exercises were usually lighter than the ones I just mentioned. Then, just as I had done ten years earlier, I decided to pull a few deadlifts one day. I deadlifted 617 pounds that day (285 kilos), and then tried it again three weeks later and pulled 650 pounds (295 kilos). This was almost a one hundred pound increase over my previous best of 555 pounds.

Now, a one hundred pound increase in the deadlift over a span of ten years is not amazing. That increase is only an average of ten pounds improvement per year. But the interesting point is that I had not pulled anything, in any manner, over 450 pounds during that time. Added to that, I had only squatted with weights around 530-540 pounds at the most. All of a sudden, a 650 pound pull was possible. Therefore, the question that arises is, "How can an athlete develop the strength to pull heavy weights without pulling heavy weights in training?" The answer, although complex, mainly lies in *repetition*. Most powerlifters deadlift once a week, with some additional auxiliary pulling exercises possibly thrown in after the deadlifts are finished. However, Olympic lifters perform a pulling movement every time they snatch, clean, RDL, snatch pull, or clean pull. Knowing that a typical Olympic lifter's training program will include several of these exercises on a daily basis, the Olympic lifter simply does many more reps of some sort of pulling exercises than the powerlifter does. Even if the Olympic lifter does not pull maximum deadlift weights every week, the pulling muscles are still being strengthened through a daily, weekly, and yearly accumulation of thousands of repetitions. This accumulated strengthening effect is what makes improved deadlift maxes possible without specializing in the deadlift.

How much ya bench?

From examining the pulling connections between power and Olympic lifting, we can move to a look at upper body strength and the bench press. And the first point that must be understood is that many successful Olympic lifters have included bench presses in their training, contrary to the usual Olympic mentality that bench pressing is a tool of Satan. IronMind training videos are available and ready for purchase that clearly show lifters like Simon Kolecki and Evgeny Chigishev bench pressing around 200 kilos. Former Canadian champion Mark Cardinal once told a story where he missed some snatch attempts at a major international competition in the 1970s, after which David Rigert told him that his upper body was not strong enough to hold the weights he was capable of pulling and that he needed to start bench pressing in training. Former Soviet world champion Gennady Ivanchenko has reported that he benched throughout his career, and the physiques of most of the great Soviet lifters of the 60s, 70s, and 80s include impressive pectoral development. My personal coach, John Thrush, benched throughout his entire Olympic lifting career and was able to clean and jerk a collegiate national record of 187.5 kilos in the 110 kilo class in 1977 while also bench pressing 480 pounds. Now, it is obviously true that many of the world's top Olympic lifters do absolutely no bench pressing at all. Nicu Vlad personally told me that he never did them. But the point here is that bench pressing is a tool of many great Olympic champions and it can be incorporated into an Olympic lifter's program with success.

Still, there is a caveat to this point. It has also become clear that bench pressing and other power/bodybuilding exercises have the potential to negatively affect upper body flexibility. If bench presses are performed with partial lock-outs, as many powerlifters do in training, the range of flexibility in the shoulder and bicep tendons will shorten and overhead lockout can suffer. I once trained a young lifter who competed in both powerlifting and Olympic lifting. With a 140 kilo clean and jerk in the 94 kilo class at eighteen years old, this athlete had obvious potential. However, he was a fanatic about the bench press and trained it much as a bodybuilder would: partial lockouts in the bench and auxiliary exercises that added tremendous upper body mass. He did go on to win a junior national championship in powerlifting, but subsequent attempts to regain his Olympic lifting skill were unsuccessful because he had simply lost his elbow lockout in the snatch and jerk. If bench pressing is going to be incorporated into an Olympic lifter's program, it must be done in a way that does not inhibit flexibility. Full el-bow lockouts in the bench and additional stretching exercises for the upper body would be useful suggestions.

Interestingly, I have also seen examples where Olympic lifting training has improved benching ability. In 1995, I trained regularly with a world powerlifting champion who was interested in Olympic lifting training just for a little variety. This athlete competed in the 165 pound class and had a top official bench press of 425 pounds, a weight he had been stuck at for three years. He dove into Olympic lifting full tilt boogie and stayed with it for around six months, drop-ping the bench press during this time. A few weeks after he decided to resume his powerlifting training, he informed me that he had bench pressed an easy 450 pounds. He told me that he could feel an obvious strength increase in his triceps and deltoids, which he attributed to the jerks and push presses he had used during his Olympic lifting time.

One other important consideration is that Olympic lifters who decide to begin bench pressing should be very careful with their pectoral tendons. Here is a personal example; I stopped bench pressing for almost eleven years, from the time I graduated high school until around 2001. I did absolutely no benching in this time. When I decided to try bench pressing again, my overall upper body strength was significantly higher. I had only bench pressed around 280 pounds in high school and by the time I decided to try them again in 2001, I had jerked 424 pounds and push pressed 319. When I resumed bench pressing, I started performing sets of five reps at around 250 pounds, which did not feel heavy at all. However, I had a string of small injuries in my pectoral tendons, mostly strains and a few partial tears. These injuries all occurred in exactly the same area, near the shoulder where the pectoral tendon connects with the humerus. They usually took around three weeks to heal with icing and no benching at all. I used bench presses in my training for around two years and I probably had five or six of these injuries. That specific part of my upper body was simply not well developed. Eventually, through gradual progressive resistance, the strength of my connective tissue caught up with the strength of my upper body muscles, the tendon injuries stopped, and I was able to bench press a mediocre 391 pounds. Did this benching improve my Olympic lifting? I would say that I noticed an increased "snappy" feeling in the lockout of my jerks. The weights felt much easier to stabilize and control when they reached arms length; I was also able to push jerk 180 kilos, which I had never done before.

Squatting? Not this time, folks...

The connections and differences between powerlifting squats and Olympic-style squats will not be discussed in this article because this subject is big enough for an article of its own. Suffice to say that a powerlifter's squats and an Olympic lifter's squats are apples and oranges, in most cases. Attempting to completely analyze this area, along with the ensuing conversation/bloodbath over whether Olympic lifters or powerlifters are stronger squatters, is like watching Chris Farley doing his Chippendale's dance on *Saturday Night Live*, with his fat rolls flapping everywhere. In other words, it can get ugly...

The great Tommy Kono once said, "If you want to be a better presser, then press." This simple statement boils down a great deal of strength training conversation to a basic truth; the best way to improve at a particular skill is to practice that skill. However, it must also be acknowledged that there are many creative variations that can enhance the performance of that skill. Vasily Alexeev used to perform clean and jerks while standing up to his chest in a river. What is the bottom line? *Simplicity and specificity are golden rules, but innovative thinking also has a place in the training of the athlete.* So before you run out and buy that "I'm an Olympic Weightlifter, so I don't bench press" t-shirt, remember that David Rigert said it was okay to bench press, and he was better than you. Many ways to skin a cat..

PUSH IT REAL GOOD:
ANOTHER LOOK AT THE SQUAT

Here is a situation for you to visualize. Many of us have probably been a part of this situation personally, and many more of us have heard hundreds of different variations of it from others. Imagine working out in a gym... any gym is possible but this is much more likely to happen in a commercial gym like Golds or 24-Hour Fitness. You are in the section of the gym where the squat racks are kept, and you are doing a squat workout. You have the bar loaded to a weight that is challenging for you... let's say that you have 315 pounds on the bar, the good old three forty-fives and a spring collar on each side. Because you were fortunate enough to have the squat taught to you properly and you've got a reasonable amount of training experience, you're using solid technique and knocking out some good deep reps. You finish your third set, put the bar back in the rack, and then you glance in the mirror and see him coming.

He has been watching you. He is wearing a tank top, leather weightlifting gloves, a gold necklace, Nike basketball shorts, an I-Pod in a Velcro pouch on his bicep, and an Oakland Raiders baseball cap (backwards). You know what's coming and you want to run, but you're not done training and you pay fifty bucks a month to work out here, so you stand your ground. When he gets to you, he mutters a few basic pleasantries and probably asks you how much you can "hit up" in the squats (his kind have their own language). It does not matter how much you tell him your best one-rep max in the squat is... 400 pounds, 800 pounds, 2,000 pounds... he will either tell you a) he has done a bigger max than you before he "jacked up" his back or b) he knows a guy who can squat between 500-700 pounds more than you. You stand and listen politely as he continues to talk about squatting but you are mentally praying that a terrorist missile will hit the building at any moment, anything to make this conversation end. Finally, he walks away and tightens up his weightlifting belt for his next set of dumbbell curls and you go back to your next set of squats.

If you have been on the receiving end of this conversation, you know how painful it is. If you have actually been the tank top/Raiders cap guy and delivered this conversation to somebody else, you should seek professional help immediately because you are directly contributing to the collapse of civilization. So why is this situation so familiar to strength athletes? Why can we all relate to it? Because the squat is one of the most controversial, debated, and lied-about exercises in the world of strength training. Thousands, possibly millions of articles and studies have been published about the squat and how it benefits the development of various types of athletes. Some people will tell you that the squat is the single best strength-building exercise that can be performed with a barbell. Other people will tell you that the squat will lead to horrible injuries. Weightlifters will tell you that powerlifting squats are phony and powerlifters will tell you that weightlifters are weak. And after all of the chalk settles, who has the magical book of truth that explains all the different aspects of the squat?

This article will not examine every facet of squatting. No single article could do that, unless it was longer than a Leo Tolstoy novel. But we should be able to cover some important territory that pertains to competitive lifters and serious strength athletes.

Technique and style

It is common knowledge that, in most cases, powerlifters and Olympic weightlifters use markedly different techniques in the squat. Olympic lifters generally squat with foot placement that is very close (or identical) to their foot placement in the receiving position of the clean and snatch. They place the bar high on the shoulders, around the base of the neck, and try to descend into the squat by pushing the knees forward and keeping the torso upright. Many people refer to this as a "high bar squat" and it is generally believed that this type of movement utilizes the quadriceps to a high degree. Incidentally, many bodybuilders squat with this style in an attempt to "isolate" their quads. Basically, an Olympic lifter's squat is designed to mimic and strengthen the positions that the body will utilize during the competition lifts. It is an assistance exercise that functions to improve the snatch and clean and jerk, and the squat technique of most lifters will look roughly the same.

Powerlifters, on the other hand, train the squat as one of their primary competition lifts and different styles will be quite noticeable. There are a variety of powerlifting squat techniques that are all intended to handle the biggest weights possible. Powerlifters will generally place the bar lower on their shoulders than Olympic lifters, sometimes tucking the bar into the "notch" where the deltoids connect with the trapezius muscles. They will usually descend into the squat by "sitting back," where the bodyweight is shifted to the heels of the foot, the shins are kept perpendicular to the floor, and the torso leans forward. This technique is often called a "low-bar squat" and is designed to utilize more of the muscles of the posterior chain, such as the hamstrings, glutes, and spinal erectors. The basic idea here is that distributing the weight of the bar among a wider range of muscle groups will allow the athlete to achieve heavier maxes. Foot placement will vary greatly from lifter to lifter. Some powerlifters, such as the great Steve Goggins and many top Europeans, use a narrow stance with their feet right around shoulder-width. But many others use a wide stance, as with the lifters of Louie

Simmons' Westside Barbell club. An athlete's body proportions, flexibility range, and personal comfort will determine which style is most effective. There is no one single correct method.

Depth is obviously a massive factor in the discussion between Olympic and powerlifting squats. Powerlifters only need to squat low enough to satisfy their competition judging requirements and, interestingly, different federations have different standards of legal depth. Generally speaking, powerlifters have to squat to a position where the thigh is roughly parallel to the floor. Squatting to this depth will only develop the flexibility of the muscles and connective tissue within the range of the movement. This is exactly why so many powerlifters have flexibility problems when they attempt to convert over to full-depth squats. Olympic lifters, however, have to utilize the squat in the same range of motion as the snatch and clean. In other words, full squat depth has to be achieved. Yet here is where it must be acknowledged that some Olympic lifters, in an effort to squat with the biggest weights possible, do not reach maximum depth when they squat. They "squat high." When this happens, there are possible performance problems that can surface. The athlete who squats high can still achieve improved lower body strength, but the transfer of that strength into the competition lifts will not be optimal. The athlete will be able to handle heavier weights in the squat because of the reduced depth and the resulting leg strength will benefit the snatch and clean and jerk, but that benefit will not be as great as the athlete who squats using full depth. I have spoken with several athletes throughout my career who have disproportionate gaps between their squat strength and their clean and jerk results. For example, I knew an athlete years ago who told me that his squats had been going well in training and that he had recently back squatted 250 kilos for six reps. But in the competition, he clean and jerked 170 kilos. This type of disparity obviously brings into question how correctly he was squatting. Also, high squatting for an Olympic lifter can increase the risk of injury because the connective tissue of the lower body will not be developed to the same degree to which it will be stretched during a maximum clean or snatch.

So who is stronger... Olympic lifters or powerlifters?

This question is the dead horse of all dead horses. I have read internet squatting arguments between powerlifters and Olympic lifters where the hostility was so intense that the argument ended with somebody mentioning that he had a concealed weapons permit and would be willing to shoot anybody who disagreed with him. All of this bickering could be solved by simply acknowledging that there are too many variables and differences between the two sports to accurately compare them. Some of the world records being established in powerlifting are phenomenal. Several superheavyweight lifters, such as Andy Bolton and Brent Mikesell, have officially squatted over 1,100 pounds. Women have officially squatted over 700 pounds. Athletes in the 165 and 181 pound bodyweight classes have officially squatted between 870 and 900 pounds and these numbers have been skyrocketing over the old records of fifteen years ago. Admittedly, there are some important factors to consider in this discussion, including completely unchecked drug use in many federations, depth judging that is lax almost to the point of non-existence, and supportive equipment such as quadruple-ply canvas slingshot squat suits that can add 300 pounds to a lifter's one-rep max. Meanwhile, Olympic lifters continue to do their squats wearing cotton gym shorts and a pair of shoes, squatting to full depth at the end of a difficult workout with no spotters or assistance. And even using this approach, some of the world's top Olympic lifters have been able to reach incredible squat weights. Soviet World Superheavyweight Champions Alexander Kurlovich and Leonid Taranenko had back squats of 350 kilos (771 pounds) and 380 kilos (837 pounds), respectively. Turkey's Dursun Sevinc, a lifter in the 85 kilo (187 pound) bodyweight class, could front squat 285 kilos (628 pounds). Therefore, could these top Olympic lifters beat the world's top powerlifters if they squatted the way powerlifters do? Or could the world's top powerlifters beat the top Olympic lifters if they took off their equipment and squatted to full depth? There are no definitive answers to these questions and this article will not delve into a guessing game.

Here is some ever-faithful personal experience to use as food for thought. I have trained the squat as both an Olympic lifter and a powerlifter. From 2001-2002, I was dabbling back and forth between the two sports and here are some findings. My best Olympic-style squat during this time was 255 kilos/562 pounds (high-bar, full depth, no supportive equipment). Within a few months of this squat, I converted to a pseudo-powerlifting squat. I moved the bar further down on my shoulders and squatted using more of a "sitting back" position with perpendicular shins and forward torso lean. My foot placement stayed exactly the same as my Olympic squat and I continued to squat to full depth. I practiced the squat this way for approximately eight weeks and bought some supportive powerlifting equipment during that time as well. When I decided to try one-rep maxes (1RM), my results were as follows: 1RM squat with a belt only- 275 kilos (606 pounds), 1RM squat with belt and knee wraps- 300 kilos (661 pounds), 1RM squat with belt, knee wraps, and Inzer squat suit- 324.5 kilos (714 pounds). The squat suit I used was loose; I was able to put it on myself in three minutes and I wore the straps down. Therefore, from slightly changing my technique and adding just the bare minimum powerlifting equipment, I was able to improve my squat from 562 pounds to 714 pounds in a short period of time (152 pounds). Many world class powerlifters have told me that 152 pounds is merely a fraction of how much supportive equipment can add if you really maximize it. I would not hesitate to guess that if I would have bought one of the mega-powered squat suits and squatted to higher depth, the 1RM would have jumped considerably.

General Strength Training and Injuries

Many athletes across the world use some form of squatting to improve their athletic performance. Football, volleyball, track and field, basketball, and various other sports teams incorporate squats into their training programs because of the obvious benefits of lower body strength, core strength, jumping ability, speed, bone density, etc. Not every sport trains the squat with the same intensity as Olympic Weightlifting, nor do they need to. But despite the demands of the sport or the degree to which the squat will be used, proper technique and weight selection is of the utmost importance because these are the keys to injury prevention.

It is possible to get injured while squatting. It is also possible to get injured while jogging, swimming, cycling, playing football, playing basketball, playing soccer, golfing, cheerleading, or typing. During any form of physical activity, the body can sustain some damage. One of the comical aspects of American sports culture is that there are certain sports which are viewed as significantly more dangerous than others, but that view is usually backwards. Almost every parent I have ever introduced to Olympic Weightlifting has an immediate cringing reaction followed by something that sounds like, "Jeez, that looks so dangerous." They see Olympic Weightlifting as being a bone-popping, ligament-snapping slaughterhouse where their children will be crippled for life. But they have no hesitation about letting their kids join football teams. Then, when fifteen year-old little Johnny blows out his ACL in football practice, everyone just shrugs and says, "It's part of the game." I coach football for a living and I have seen more injuries in two seasons of football than I have seen in twenty years of weightlifting.

Vigorous physical activity carries the potential for danger. That is simply something that must be understood. Tiger Woods had to limp through the US Open last year on a knee that had been injured from golf! Marathon runners battle hip bursitis and plica syndrome. Gymnasts slip on the uneven bars and crash face first into the ground. On and on it goes. But for a variety of reasons, deep squatting movements are still thought by many people to be excessively dangerous. The truth, which is verified through years and years of experience from thousands of weightlifters, is that injuries from deep squatting movements are extraordinarily rare if the athlete uses the proper combination of stretching, solid technique, sensible weight selection, warming up, and post-workout recovery. The health and performance benefits far outweigh the risks. If you don't want to risk getting hurt, it might be wise to select a pastime that involves less squatting. Drag racing might be a more suitable choice, where you are only one gas leak away from a fiery car explosion that will send you into a brick wall at two hundred miles per hour.

Back to the guy with the Raiders cap...

The squat is practically worshiped by many strength enthusiasts. Dale Clark's famous poem "The Squat" is plastered on the walls of gyms all across the country, concluding with the immortal line "...the trouble with you is you ain't been SQUATTIN!" Pages of cartoons have been drawn that ridicule the typical flamingo-workout physique, where the guy struts across the gym with his massive pecs and biceps and legs that look like a pair of plyers with shorts on. Some people love the squat, but some people fear it. For the last few years, a photograph has been circulating around the global e-mail network of a powerlifter that supposedly blew his internal organs out through his anus by pushing too hard on a squat. The picture is a phony that was doctored to look that way, but the terror is still out there. It has always been my opinion that the fear associated with the squat is caused by the simple fact that squatting is hard work. Most people don't want to do things that require massive levels of strain and exertion. It is much easier to simply dismiss it as dangerous, and the exaggerations of the danger can be amazingly bizarre. When I was working out in high school, a coach once told me about an athlete who had attempted a squat that was too heavy for him and it caused his patella to burst out of his skin and fly across the room like it had been shot out of a cannon. These are Boogeyman stories, but the guy with the Raiders cap believes every word of them. This is why it is important for weightlifters and serious strength athletes to develop a thick skin about it and, if possible, find a place to train where everyone understands that mastering the squat is the law of the land.

FATTIES

This morning, I was watching an old video of the 1998 European Championships in my living room. My wife had our other TV on in the bedroom and she was watching the Today Show. I overheard a segment on the show about how childhood obesity has become such a huge problem in our country that many parents are hiring personal fitness trainers for their kids because their kids are already fat by the time they're 10-12 years old. While I applaud the effort to fight childhood obesity, I guess the question that pops into my mind is, "How did the parents allow these kids to live an early lifestyle that led them to obesity at 10 years old?" And then, as I'm watching a bunch of European lifters snatching 170 at 85, 150 at 69, etc., I think to myself, "I wonder if their parents hired fitness trainers to combat their childhood obesity when they were growing up in Bulgaria?" American kids often grow up soft, lazy, flabby, and weak because our society has become so consumed by technology and EASE. Many kids just don't grow up tough anymore in the US. I'd be willing to bet that a lot of these top lifters from Europe, especially the ones who grow up in countries like Bulgaria, had to fight through a lot of adversity in their early years. This doesn't mean that making our kids dig ditches in the back yard for eight hours a day during their pre-teen years is going to solve all of our sport and social problems, but it couldn't hurt anything.

GET UP, STAND UP: THE SPIRITUAL PRINCIPLES OF SQUATTING

When I look back at the *Performance Menu* articles I've been writing in recent months, I notice that several of them have dealt with topics such as coaching philosophy, mental strength, team building, etc. They've been fun to write and I definitely still have a lot to say about all of these areas, but I think it's time to break things up and make this month's article specifically dedicated to a training topic. Everybody who reads this magazine (as far as I know) is some kind of strength athlete, and most of you probably use the Olympic lifts as some component of your training life.

And that's why we're going to go back to the basics this month and take another look at SQUATTING. I wrote a PM article about squatting once, many moons ago, but it mostly focused on the technique differences between high-bar and low-bar squats. This month, we're going to analyze squats as they apply to athletes who focus specifically on the Olympic lifts. I've wanted to revisit this topic for a long time because, in a nutshell, squatting is absolutely one of the most important tools in the training of any type of strength athlete. If you're an Olympic lifter, powerlifter, strongman competitor, bodybuilder, shotputter, general barbell trainer, etc., then squatting has to be part of your basic belief system. You have to believe in squatting the same way a Christian missionary believes in the Ten Commandments. Just like the missionary relies on his biblical principles to guide him through life's struggles, you have to rely on squatting to get you through the tough times of your quest for strength. When everything else has failed you, you still have squatting. Squats will never fail you. If you do them, you will get results. Your body will be strong. If you can't squat because of injury, disability, or lack of motivation, you will end up with nothing. The most important muscles of your body will shrink and you will eventually become weak. You'll be like a formerly dedicated religious zealot who has lost his way and drifted into a sea of drugs and hookers. You must be washed clean through surgery, rehab, mental re-commitment or whatever else needs to be done to put you back on the road to strength righteousness. It will be a baptism by fire, because hard squatting isn't exactly designed for your comfort. But the pain is just something you'll have to accept. If you want things to be easy, you might want to read another magazine.

Open your hymnals, brothers and sisters. It's time to read the scriptures. We're going to take a look at five basic principles of squatting that will steer you in the right direction, if you follow them. Feel free to shout hallelujah, speak in tongues, or be slain in the spirit at any moment.

The First Principle: Squatting is the most important assistance exercise in Olympic lifting, but it is still an assistance exercise. Squatting proficiency cannot be undervalued for athletes who want to improve in the snatch and clean and jerk. Both of the full competitive movements obviously involve a squat phase, and it is impossible to achieve maximum results in these lifts if squats are not being used in training because the benefits in overall body strength are impossible to replicate with any other assistance lift. Some people view the squat as a lower body lift, but there is much more benefit than simply what happens in the muscles of the legs. Squatting is one of the best core exercises in existence. The postural muscles of the abdomen, spinal erectors, obliques, and even the middle/upper back will be strengthened every time a squat is performed. The rewards of the squat exceed those of any other barbell exercise, plain and simple.

However, it's important to understand the place of the squat in the training of an Olympic lifter. The squat is the finest assistance exercise available, but it is still an assistance exercise. Sometimes I think American Olympic lifters get carried away with squat enthusiasm and they start to believe that heavier squatting will fix anything. Their philosophy becomes, "Squatting will make you a better snatcher. Squatting will make you a better cleaner. Squatting will make you a better jerker." This type of thinking has good intentions because it shows respect to the squat as being hugely important. But there is a caveat here. Olympic lifters often get so focused on bigger squat numbers that they will start squatting incorrectly to get them. The depth starts to get shallow, the torso starts to lean forward, knee wraps come out, etc. All of these things start to happen because the lifter is obsessed with getting bigger squat weights, but none of them will translate into the movements of the snatch or clean. If you are an Olympic lifter, you have to always understand that the squat's purpose is to make you stronger for the Olympic lifts. This means that the technique and positions of the squat have to stay as close as possible to the technique and positions of the snatch and clean. If you want to become a better snatcher, correctly practicing the snatch is the best way to do it. Squatting will make you stronger, and that strength will give you a better chance to snatch more weight. But the squats have to be used correctly if there is going to be any carryover to the competition lifts. When I was doing my best lifting, one of my close competitors had a one-rep max in the squat that was twenty kilos heavier than mine. But in competition, I could stand up with a 180 kilo clean easier than he could. Who was using the squat most effectively in training?

The Second Principle: Front Squats are a "position lift." Because of the basic movement of the clean and jerk, Olympic lifters use the front squat as an essential training tool. In fact, there are some voices in the weightlifting community who believe that front squats are more important than back squats. Much of this philosophy comes from the perception of the Bulgarian program. Several outsiders have mistakenly believed that the Bulgarians only use front squats in their training, no back squats. As I said, this is not the case. But the idea still lingers on message boards, forums, etc. Regardless, front squats are one of the primary weapons of the Olympic lifter. Everyone agrees to this.

One of the reasons why front squats are so beneficial is the upper body strength gains that accompany the movement. That's right... front squats are as much an upper body strength movement as they are a lower body strength movement. When I started training for the Calpian weightlifting club in the early 90s, coach John Thrush explained to me that front squats are a "position lift." This means that they are used not just to strengthen the muscles of the legs, but also the muscles of the upper body that hold the barbell on the shoulders in the receiving position of the clean. When an athlete performs a clean or a front squat, the muscles of the chest, shoulders, arms, and upper back are used to maintain the proper form of the movement (keeping the elbows high, the chest expanded, the shoulders wide, etc.) Heavy front squatting develops the stabilizing strength of these muscles, even though the arms and shoulders are basically immobile throughout the lift.

This is why it is imperative that the lifter performs the front squat with exactly the same upper body position as the clean. There will be no upper body strength development if the front squats are performed in the sloppy manner we have all seen at some point (shoulders rounding forward, elbows dropping, fingers popping off the bar, etc.) A small amount of this technical sloppiness might occur when an athlete is pushing for a new one-rep max in the front squat. That's understandable. But letting incorrect upper body positions become a regular part of your front squat technique will limit the benefits of the lift, and also increase the chance for injury.

The Third Principle: Stop Squats... A misunderstood ally. Stop squats are not difficult to explain. A stop squat is a high-bar, Olympic style back squat with a one-second pause at the bottom. Some people refer to these as "pause squats" but "stop squat" is the name I use. I don't think there are many weightlifting coaches or athletes who use stop squats as a regular part of their training. And I don't understand this, because the rewards are tremendous. I have used stop squats throughout every phase of my serious weightlifting career, and also with every serious lifter I have ever coached. All of these lifters have done the best lifts of their careers while using stop squats. When I was doing the best lifting of my life, I used my top stop squat triple as the barometer of how strong I was. In other words, the heaviest weight I could do a set of three with in training told me how ready I was for a big clean and jerk.

People sometimes misunderstand the purpose of stop squats. I was reading a discussion on the internet recently where a group of lifters were explaining how the main purpose of the stop squat was to prepare an athlete to recover from a botched clean. Because of the pause at the bottom of the stop squat, the lift resembles a heavy clean where the athlete gets "planted" in the bottom of the clean and has to pause or double-bounce before standing up. Let me make it clear that stop squats are not intended to improve the athlete's performance of an incorrect clean. It might be one of the residual benefits of stop squats that the athlete has more reserve strength for standing up from a paused clean, but that is not the primary purpose. Stop squats are a valuable exercise for two reasons. 1) The pause at the bottom of the squat forces the athlete to maintain total muscle contraction with a heavy weight on the shoulders, which increases the stabilizer strength of the athlete's torso. 2) The lack of rebound momentum prior to standing up from the squat forces the muscles of the lower body to push harder to complete the lift, which increases the potential power output of the entire body. But don't take my word for it. The proof is in the pudding. Incorporate stop squats into your lifting program and you will get stronger. So let it be written.

The Fourth Principle: Sets and Reps... The possibilities are endless. How often should an Olympic lifter train the squats? How many sets and reps should be performed in a typical workout? How often should new one-rep maxes be attempted? In other words, how in the hell should you implement the squats into your training program to improve your lifts?

I've said this many times in the past, but there are several different ways to train the squat effectively. Nobody has the one magical answer. Throughout my years as a lifter, I've probably seen at least fifty different types of set/rep programs, and many of them have had outstanding results. My personal preference is as follows:

How many times per week should the athlete squat? Three. One front squat workout, one back squat workout, and one stop squat workout. The best days to do them are Monday, Thursday, and Saturday. Friday and Sunday will always be off days, and Tuesday will always be a relatively light workout.

What kind of sets and reps should be used? Sets of three reps (triples) are always reliable for an Olympic lifter. I'm an old-school lifter, so I have always liked the old 3x3 method. This means that the athlete performs three or four warm-up sets before picking the "target weight" for that workout and doing three sets of three with it. Now, variety is always going to have some benefits. I have never used sets higher than five reps when training competitive lifters, but that's just the method I prefer. There are other accomplished coaches who use sets of 8-10 reps with their lifters. One of our top American coaches has a volume phase for his lifters where the athletes are doing sets of ten reps in squats, pulls, push presses, and other assistance exercises. I don't think any Olympic lifting coaches would stay with this many reps throughout the entire competition year, but using high-rep sets during a "volume phase" can lead to positive results for some athletes.

How often should Olympic lifters attempt new one-rep maxes? Not often. And when the athlete does attempt a new 1RM, it would be wise to do it at a time when it won't negatively affect the athlete's snatching and clean and jerking. Planning those squat max-out sessions around the same time when the athlete is attempting heavy attempts in the SN or C&J can get dicey.

The Fifth Principle: Bigger squats = Better snatches, true or false? An athlete can improve their leg strength without moving up their one-rep squat max. It's true, it's true. Let me give you a personal example to illustrate this. When I was twenty, my best squat was 500 pounds at around 215 bodyweight. I did this squat at the beginning of a workout when I was totally fresh, I wore light knee wraps, the bar was sitting low on my shoulders, my depth was around parallel, and there was a lot of forward lean with the torso. My best snatch was 120 kilos and best clean and jerk was 150.

Shortly after this 500 pound squat, I changed coaches and my training program became completely different. After one year, I maxed out in the squat and did 217.5 kilos (479 pounds) at 218 bodyweight. I did this squat at the end of a hard workout, I wore nothing on my knees, the bar was sitting high up at the base of my neck, I sat down to 100% full depth, and my torso basically stayed straight up and down. This squat max was 21 pounds lower than the 500 pound squat I had done a year earlier. At this time, my best snatch was 135 kilos and my best clean and jerk was 167.5.

The point here is that the athlete's leg strength and overall power output can increase simply by squatting in a stricter, more technically disciplined manner. Making your squats sloppier and higher for the sake of a few more kilos will not make you a better Olympic lifter. Adding new kilos to your squat max while maintaining perfect technique in the squats will translate into stronger competition lifts. The athletes (and the coaches) have to be perfectionists about squat form.

Amen, brothers and sisters. Now you have five random principles about squatting that will absolutely, positively make you a better Olympic lifter if you decide to make them part of your training life. If you implement all of these ideas into your training and your total doesn't go up, please contact Greg Everett for a refund on your *Performance Menu* subscription. I don't think you'll have much to worry about though, because regardless of exactly which squatting approach you decide to use in your training, everybody needs to follow some of the same basic rules. He who has eyes to see, let him see. He who has eyes to hear, let him hear.

ONE AND ONE AND ONE IS THREE... AND OTHER COMPLICATED IDEAS ABOUT POWER SNATCHES

A couple of nights ago, I was sitting in a bar with my wife and some friends of ours. We were listening to a band that played mostly classic rock from the late sixties and seventies (my kind of stuff) and this group had their act nailed down tight. The best moment of their show was when they tore through "Come Together" by the Beatles, which is a song that most of the smart people in the world probably love. I had already enjoyed a good steak and sampled plenty of Ireland's finest beverage specialties, and this song made me start thinking about weightlifting. That might sound odd, but I probably never go more than thirty or forty waking minutes without thinking about weightlifting in my normal life anyway. So thinking about snatches while I'm listening to John Lennon's lyrics about spinal crackers isn't all that unusual for me.

The title of this song made me think about all the different physical qualities that have to "come together" to make an Olympic lift work properly. Over the last few months, I've been visiting a lot of different gyms and teaching snatches, cleans, and jerks to some great people who want to master these lifts. Most of these athletes have already learned the basics of the power snatch and power clean before I get there and start working with them. This is obviously helpful because the power snatch and power clean allow the learner to practice the pulling movements of the lifts without worrying about the challenging transition that takes place when the lifter has to perform the full lifts and take those snatches and cleans down to the bottom position.

However, this particular subject takes me to the topic of this month's article. If you've spent some time in the Olympic lifts, you probably know that some weightlifters continue to use the power snatch and power clean as part of their training programs even throughout their intermediate and advanced stages. What I want to look at this month is the value of this. *In other words, should weightlifters continue to spend time doing power snatches and power cleans in their training once they've passed the beginner stages and learned the full versions of the snatch and clean?* I've actually wanted to write an article about this subject for several months because I know there are a lot of different opinions about it. So you can thank The Harry McGraw Band and Irish Car Bombs for finally bringing this idea to paper.

What are Power Snatches and Power Cleans?

I always assume *Performance Menu* readers have a solid level of previous weight-lifting knowledge when I write these articles each month, but let's just quickly make sure we all know what we're talking about before we get too far into this discussion. A power snatch/clean is basically just a snatch or clean where the athlete catches the bar overhead and does not sit down into the full squat bottom position. Power snatches and power cleans are usually caught in approximately a quarter-squat position.

Right away, I need to throw in my personal opinion about these lifts. Over the years, I've heard some athletes and coaches who have different definitions of what a power snatch/clean is. The idea they use is that power snatches/cleans are determined by the depth of the squat position when the athlete catches the bar in the receiving position, but they judge these lifts the way a powerlifting referee judges squat depth. The idea is, "If the lifter has to squat below parallel to complete the lift, it's not a power snatch. If the squat position doesn't break parallel, it's a power snatch." I don't like this idea because I think a legitimate power snatch/clean takes place when the lifter completes the lift with only a few degrees of knee bend. When the weight gets heavy enough that the lifter has to squat "around parallel" before standing up and finishing the lift, it's not a true power snatch/clean. At this point, the lift becomes a kind of almost-a-full-snatch-but-not-really type of thing. I simply prefer to have clearer distinctions between power movements and full movements, so this is the way I look at it.

Moving on, I think most coaches in the world probably include the power snatch/clean in the earliest teaching phase when working with new athletes. I definitely do. The transition into a full bottom position of a snatch or clean is athletically demanding, and newbies usually need to learn how to power snatch/clean before they start moving on to learning the complete movements with deep receiving positions. Athletes who use the Olympic lifts to improve their perfor-mance in a different sport, such as football or track and field, often stick to the power snatch/clean in their workouts full-time because the primary reason they use the Olympic lifts at all is to reap the benefits of the triple-extension pulling movement, and sitting down into a deep receiving position simply isn't necessary for them to accomplish what they want. However, this article focuses on athletes who are either A) competitive Olympic lifters or B) strength athletes who want to improve in the full versions of the Olympic lifts.

An important question that pops up is "Why would any weightlifters con-tinue to use the power snatch/clean in training after they have learned to perform the full movements?" I'll try to give you a short combination of answers I've heard for this question from different people over the years. One of the first answers is that the power snatch/clean provides variety in training, and the benefit is that the athlete simply doesn't get mentally burned out from constantly doing the full lifts. Another answer I've heard is that the power snatch/clean builds up greater explosive pulling power because the higher receiving position forces the athlete to elevate the barbell higher than in a full snatch/clean, so the nature of the power snatch/clean demands a snappy full extension of the top pull. I've also heard some coaches say that the power snatch/clean prevents some of the pounding on the knees that occurs when athletes perform full movements, so the joints of the lower body get some rest from the constant strain of maximum-depth lifts.

Now, the Mang Foremong Version...

So these are some of the reasons why weightlifting athletes would continue to incorporate the power snatch/clean into their training programs after they've already learned and, at least to some degree, mastered the full versions of the lifts. However, this is where I need to make some statements. I personally do not believe that the power snatch/clean is particularly valuable to an experienced weightlifter. There is no way that I would ever issue a complete condemnation of them, nor would I ever say, "Power snatches and power cleans are a waste of time unless you're a beginner." It's impossible to make a statement like that because there are some very high-level athletes and coaches who use them (I'll mention a few examples later).

But my experience in weightlifting has led me to think that the best way to perfect the technique of the full snatch/clean is simply to practice the full movements, along with pulls and squats. From a personal perspective, I can tell you that from 1993 through 1998, I went from a 115 kilo snatch to a 155 kilo snatch and I know for certain that I did not use power snatches in my training at all during this time. I also went from a 155 kilo clean to a 187.5 kilo clean during this same time period, but I did use power cleans on a semi-regular basis in training. The power clean, in my opinion, has a slightly more beneficial translation to the full clean than the power snatch has to the full snatch.

One of the main reasons why I don't like using power snatches/cleans for experienced weightlifters is the problem of foot positioning in the turnover. Most weightlifters lift their feet from the platform and jump them outwards when they are making the transition from the pull to the receiving position. Some coaches call this "jumping the feet from the pull stance to the squat stance" or some other terminology. Some athletes, such as superheavyweight world snatch record holder Behdad Salimi, lift their feet several inches from the platform and then jump them into the squat receiving position with a loud SLAP on the platform. Other athletes, such as former superheavyweight Olympic champion Alexander Kurlovich, lift the feet only as much as necessary for re-positioning into their squat, so the feet look like they're almost "sliding" outwards. Regardless of the amount of lift from the platform, almost all successful lifters jump their feet laterally into their squat width when turning over the lifts. Here is where I notice a problem with the power snatch/clean.

Almost all of the lifters I've seen in my life jump their feet out to the sides at least a few inches wider when they perform power snatches/cleans than they do when they practice the full lifts. In other words, the turnover of the power snatch/clean is different from the turnover of the full snatch/clean because the athlete is probably lifting the feet from the platform and moving them out much wider than usual during the power movements. This is done because when an athlete is performing a power snatch/clean with any significant weight on the bar, the athlete has to get into a lower position in the turnover to be able to successfully complete the lift. If the athletes know that the lift is supposed to be a power snatch/clean, then they are going to try to complete the lift with minimum knee bend in the receiving position. In order to get lower under the bar and lock out the lift overhead AND maintain minimum knee bend, the body's only biomechanical option is to move the feet out to a wider position. If any of you have done heavy power snatches/cleans yourselves or worked with anybody who does them, you probably know exactly what I'm talking about. I've seen some lifters attempt maximum weights in the power snatch/clean where they jump their feet out so wide that the lift looks like an ultra-wide stance powerlifting squat.

As I see it, there are a few potential problems here. First of all, the injury risk increases when the athlete attempts heavy power snatches/cleans with excessively wide foot placement in the turnover. As we mentioned before, some coaches like power snatches/cleans because the joints of the lower body are relieved of some of the pounding that takes place when attempting full lifts with maximum-depth receiving positions. But if the athletes are doing power snatches/cleans with excessively wide foot placement, the risk of groin pulls and ankle strains becomes more significant. Second of all (and this is the main problem I see with power snatches/cleans), the muscle memory of the full movements is not being fully developed. I believe that the best way to improve in the Olympic lifts is for the athlete to practice thousands upon thousands of perfect, identical full snatches and cleans. This way, the motor patterns of the lifts become so deeply ingrained in the athlete's neurological system that the athlete's body simply doesn't know how to do an incorrect lift. This type of "muscle memorization" becomes less likely when the athlete is continually going back and forth between power snatches/cleans and full snatches/cleans.

So when I coach athletes (and in my own lifting career), I do no power snatches at all, and only some moderate power clean workouts early in the competition training cycle. When a competition or a max-out session is approaching, the lifter is only practicing the full lifts.

There's always a big asterisk next to everything...

Now that I've taken a definitive stance on this issue and asserted my opinion with clear reasoning, let me tell you about a few noteworthy examples that basically contradict most of what I just said.

As I mentioned in a *Performance Menu* article from a few years ago, I trained with Olympic Champion Nicu Vlad for a month back in 1990 when he was still one of the top lifters in the world. Vlad is one of the greatest snatchers in history, with a record of 441 pounds in the old 220 pound bodyweight class. By any standard, he is one of the great lifters of all time. And Vlad used a lot of power snatches in his workouts. In fact, he used the power snatch in one of the most interesting ways I've ever seen. When doing a snatch workout, Vlad would power snatch most of the lighter weights of his warm-up. As the weights got progressively heavier from set to set, his receiving position would get incrementally deeper and deeper. His foot positioning was identical every time, and he had none of the excessive-width power snatch foot placement problems that I described above. His power snatches would simply hit a deeper receiving position as he snatched 90 kilos, 110 kilos, 130 kilos, 150 kilos, etc. By the time he was loading up 180 kilos on the bar, he was performing full snatches. In twenty-three years of weightlifting, I've never seen an athlete with as much control over their body as Vlad had. He controlled his body the way Ray Charles controlled the piano.

Another example is 1996 Olympic Champion Pablo Lara from Cuba. Lara was the top lifter in the world in the old 76 kilo class (177 lbs), with a 205 kilo (451 lbs) clean and jerk. You read that right... 177 bodyweight and a 451 clean and jerk. In the Atlanta training hall before the '96 Games, Lara did some of the most impressive power cleans I have ever seen. In one workout that he did less than a week before he competed, he power clean and jerked 190 kilos (418 lbs). It looked like just another routine training lift for Lara, and it was mechanically identical to the rest of his lifts. None of the potential technical glitches that I described earlier were present in his lifts.

To summarize our discussion, Matt Foreman says that power snatches/ cleans are not especially beneficial to an experienced weightlifter, but some of the best lifters in the world use them in training. Yeah, that sounds about right. So let me give you a few final thoughts that should tie all of this together and keep me from looking like a mental midget. First of all, what I've described in this article is my own personal philosophy on power snatches/cleans. You can simply add it to the library of training philosophies you're accumulating in your mind as you learn about this sport. I have over two decades of experience in weightlifting and I've had a successful career at the national level, so I guess I can humbly say that my opinions didn't just fall off a turnip truck. However, there are obviously other well-credentialed people in the sport who have slightly different philosophies than mine.

Keep a couple of things in mind, though. Power snatches and cleans have some potential shortcomings, as we described above. But athletes like Vlad and Lara have found a way to incorporate power movements into their training without letting those shortcomings emerge. In other words, Vlad uses power snatches but he doesn't have foot placement problems in the full lifts. Why is this? Well, one of the main reasons is that Vlad is an extremely exceptional athlete. As I have written in the past, some athletes are able to take kinesthetic awareness to a higher level. He is one of them. The technique hazards that many of us have to work hard to overcome simply don't apply to Vlad. He can do a full snatch, or a power snatch to any level of depth, and his body will hit the correct positions every time.

Does this mean that we should train differently than Vlad because we have to start by openly admitting that he's a better athlete than any of us? No, not necessarily. I think it's important to study the training methods of world champions and then use those methods to make yourself better. The main point of this discussion is that most of you who are reading this article are probably in the beginning/intermediate stages of your weightlifting careers. Because of this, it's important that you understand the benefits and hazards that go along with every aspect of your training. If you can utilize power snatches to make you a better athlete the way Nicu Vlad has done, then go for it. But you should design them into your training program with a clear idea about which technical qualities you want to develop and which ones you DON'T want to develop.

Let's finish it off by looking at it this way. The Beatles started their career by saying, "She loves you... yeah, yeah, yeah." They finished their career by saying, "He got feet down below his knees, hold you in his arms till you can feel his disease." In other words, they started pretty basic and they got more complex as they practiced and gained experience (and dropped acid). If you handle your weightlifting career the same way (minus the acid), you might wind up with fame, money, and a relatively hot one-legged wife. Happy hunting.

LET YOUR FREAK FLAG FLY

When I first got started in Olympic Weightlifting, a very thoughtful coach was nice enough to give me a couple of VHS video tapes with tons of weightlifting footage on them. He knew I was interested in becoming a weightlifter and he wanted to help me out, so he told me to take these tapes home and learn as much as I could from them. One of the tapes was an old weightlifting instructional video that was put together by the USWF (you're showing your age when you recognize that abbreviation). I believe our former National Coaching Director Gene Baker was the narrator of the video and it was extremely helpful to me as I tried to learn the sport. In the video, a coach went through the standard teaching progression of the snatch, clean, jerk, and various assistance movements. There were several athletes who performed the Olympic lifts in the videos and I was blown away by how sharp and efficient their lifts were. Their technique mirrored the sequence photos I had seen on posters and in magazines. Their lifts looked exactly the way they were supposed to, according to everything I had learned. They had the proper starting position off the floor with flat backs and straight arms, they accelerated smoothly through the first and second pull, they kept their shoulders over the bar, they extended straight and shrugged hard at the top of the movement, etc. They were masters of what you might call "standard technique." Remember that phrase: "standard technique."

The other video the coach gave me was a collection of championship meets. One of the meets that was on the tape was the 1988 Olympics in Seoul. I probably watched this tape a thousand times (I still have it, by the way), and obviously the highlight of the whole show was Naim Suleymanoglu of Turkey, who won the gold medal in the old 60 kilo weight class with a 152.5 kilo snatch and 190 kilo clean and jerk. For those of you who don't speak in kilos, that's a 132 pound man who snatched 336 pounds and clean and jerked 418. Think about those numbers for a second.

Naim's performance baffled me for a couple of reasons. First of all, it was difficult to understand how a man that size could lift those weights. I still don't think the world has totally grasped it. But second, I was confused by Naim's lifting because his technique was very, very different from the "standard technique" I had learned on the coaching video. Naim jerked the weights off the floor, his pull speed looked like a grinding max deadlift, he tilted his torso backwards at the top of his second pull, his turnover was like a rocket, his feet were set unevenly prior to his jerk dip, and then he seemed to lunge forward as he was splitting under the bar in the jerk. This wasn't standard technique. This was freak-of-the-week technique, and he was lifting world records with it.

The confusion here is also the subject of this article. We're going to talk about freaks. Or more concisely, we're going to talk about world class athletes who smash records and win gold medals despite the fact that they drastically deviate from the normal, accepted technique of the Olympic lifts. When we use the phrase "standard technique" in this article, we're talking about the classic, by-the-book technical models that all of us have probably learned through working with a coach, watching videos, studying sequence photos, etc. This standard technique approach is what almost every coach in the world uses to teach beginners, so how in the hell does it come to pass that certain athletes can modify this technique and then go on to beat everyone on the planet?

I'll answer this question at the end of the article, brothers and sisters. But first, let's take a look at a few of weightlifting's greatest freaks and what it is that makes them so... you know, freaky.

That's Mister Dimas, to you...

Pyrros Dimas of Greece is one of the most successful weightlifters in history. This man won three Olympic gold medals and was one jerk away from winning four. In addition to having this phenomenal record, Dimas is probably the most exciting, intense weightlifter I've seen in my lifetime. Dimas lifted weights the way Jimi Hendrix played guitar. It made your blood chill to watch him in action.

But Dimas stupefied the weightlifting community for years because of his pulling technique. If you've seen this man lift, you probably already know what I'm talking about. If you haven't seen him lift, get on YouTube as soon as possible and check it out. Here's how it worked: when Dimas pulled his snatches and cleans, the bar came off the floor and passed the knees in a pretty normal fashion. But when the bar was passing his knees, Dimas would actually stretch his neck forward and then violently whip his head back as he finished his top pull. Many of us called this "the Dimas head whip." It was odd to watch. Many other lifters have pulled their heads backwards as they finished their top pulls. Pyrros was not the only one. But the way he extended his neck forward and then blasted his skull backwards as he extended his second pull was unlike anyone else.

And remarkably, this technical abnormality created no problems for him. His balance was never adversely affected. The bar stayed close to his body, he had incredible consistency, and he also managed to snatch around 180 kilos and clean around 210 throughout his career in the 85 kilo class. How could the guy lift so successfully with such a strange, abnormal technical habit?

The Old Chicken Wing Special...

Pulling with bent arms, that's what we're talking about here. I would venture a guess that almost every single weightlifting instructor in history has probably taught his/her athletes to keep their arms straight throughout the pull. One of my first coaches used to say, "Your arms are like ropes. They're just there to hang on to the bar. You pull the bar with your legs, back and traps." Okay, we get it. You might have even heard a similar piece of advice from a coach in your own weightlifting background.

So how in the heck can we explain it when we see some of the top weightlifters in the world pulling their lifts with their arms bent? Make no mistake about it, there have been some very successful lifters who have done it. Some of the greatest pound-for-pound lifts in history came from a lifter who many people have forgotten over the years, Bulgaria's Mikhail Petrov. Petrov was a world champion in the old 67.5 kilo (148 pound) weight class in the mid-eighties. This man could snatch 157.5 kilos (347 lbs) and clean and jerk 200 kilos (440 lbs) in this weight class. And yes, he pulled his lifts with his arms bent. As soon as the bar came off the floor, his elbows were cocked and they stayed that way all throughout the top of his second pull. It was a violation of every fundamental weightlifting technique lesson in the sport, but Petrov wasn't the only guilty party.

Another one of the world's greatest bent-arm pullers comes right here from the good old United States. Mario Martinez is an American legend. 1984 Olympic silver medalist, ten-time national champion, American record-holder, Pan Am Champion, and the list goes on. I was fortunate enough to compete in some of the same meets with Mario in the early nineties when I was starting my career and he was finishing his. In the superheavyweight class, Mario snatched 415 pounds and clean and jerked 518. These are phenomenal accomplishments and still, to this day, the only American who has toppled these numbers is the Oklahoma Ox, Shane Hamman. But back to Mario... he was a notorious bent-arm puller. In both the snatch and the clean, just like Mikhail Petrov, Mario's elbows were cocked before the bar even came off the ground. Both of these athletes utilized a technique deviation that no qualified weightlifting coach would allow a young athlete to do for two seconds. So once again, how could these guys lift so successfully with such a strange, abnormal technical habit?

Does a God Make Mistakes?

One of most respected and revered athletes in the history of our sport is the great Soviet Union legend Urik Vardanian. Over twenty years ago, Vardanian totaled 405 kilos in the old 82.5 kilo class. Just to put that in perspective for you newbies, the Olympic gold medals that are being won these days in the 85 kilo class are usually by way of totals in the 385-395 range. Vardanian set a standard of excellence in our sport that still stands as one of the benchmarks of weightlifting magnificence.

And technically, Vardanian was another one of those athletes who did things much differently from what we would consider normal. When Vardanian pulled the bar from the floor, his legs straightened and his hips shot up much earlier than standard technique would dictate. When the bar arrived at Vardanian's knees, his body position looked a lot like an RDL. His legs were almost completely straight and his torso was leaning forward dramatically. Any coach who had a trainee exhibit this kind of technique in the gym would probably say something like "your butt is coming up too fast." And using this kind of technique, Vardanian snatched over 400 pounds at 180 bodyweight.

He had another crazy feature in the jerk, as well. Vardanian was a split jerker, as most lifters are, but he simply did not split his feet very far. I think almost every weightlifting coach in the world would consider Vardanian's split position to be too narrow or shallow. But he used this narrow split and jerked almost 500 pounds at the same 180 bodyweight. I encourage you readers with internet access to get on YouTube and examine Urik's lifts for yourself. Many of them are available in slow motion and you will see exactly what we're talking about. All of this begs the question, how could the guy lift so successfully with such a strange, abnormal technical habit?

Okay, so?

These lifters are among the elite of our sport's history. They have mastered the Olympic lifts to a degree that almost nobody has been able to equal, and each of them demonstrated technique variations that clearly contradict the normal movement models of the snatch, clean, and jerk. How is this possible, and how does it make any sense? The answer can be explained this way.

Some athletes are phenomenally talented. They are born with very unique combinations of athleticism, strength, and kinesthetic awareness. For those of you who don't recognize that last term, kinesthetic awareness refers to an athlete's heightened understanding of his/her body's positions, strengths, and movements. People with increased kinesthetic awareness have the ability to move their bodies effectively without much coaching or instruction. As coaches, we have all worked with athletes who simply seem to "get it" much quicker than others. Some athletes need instructions, demonstrations, and literal hands-on manipulation to make their bodies move in the correct pattern; and then after all that work, they still struggle. And then other athletes can watch a skill demonstrated by someone else, listen to a few simple verbal cues, and then perform the skill with an immediate level of expertise. We all understand this. Some people have more natural ability than others.

However, athletes like Vardanian and Dimas have taken kinesthetic awareness to a higher level. These athletes have actually learned the standard technique of the Olympic lifts and then, over a long period of practice, they have customized the movements to fit their own individual strengths and proportions. They have formed their own technique the way a potter molds clay into the exact shape he wants to see. Vardanian's hip-rise technique was formed because he had very long legs. His femurs were much longer proportionately than the average athlete, and so he found a way to adapt the standard technique of the lifts in the most advantageous way for his own personal physiology. He might not have even known that he was developing his own personal technique as he practiced and trained year after year. He might have simply been performing the snatch and the clean in the way that made him most comfortable and successful. Dimas, at some point in his training youth, found that his lifts were much more explosive and effective if he whipped his head back like a wrecking ball at the top of his pull. This discovery could have been the result of an extreme strength level in the muscles in the upper back, or some other region where he was personally more developed than other athletes. I doubt if Dimas himself could explain it to you any more clearly than a bird could explain to you how it flies.

That leaves you, as coaches, in sticky territory because you have to ask yourself, "When is it okay for me to let my athletes deviate from standard technique?" If you're working with a young lifter and, somewhere during the teaching process, this lifter starts to whip his head like Dimas, should you tell the lifter not to do it? Are you stopping that lifter from using a technique deviation that could eventually make him a world champion if he masters it? There isn't an easy answer.

Athletes need quality coaching and instruction. We all understand this. However, athletes also need to be allowed some freedom at some point to develop on their own. This is the hardest thing to accept as a coach because you feel like you're not doing your job if you're not actively teaching. Letting the athlete "leave the nest" and develop on their own is a challenging thing. And I'm not saying that coaches should teach the basics to their athletes and then say, "Okay, now it's all up to you." This is abandonment, which isn't going to be productive in most cases. But I am saying that after the basic teaching and modeling has taken place, the athlete has to be allowed some leeway to practice and grow. If one of your lifters develops a technical deviation like the ones we've analyzed here, my advice would be to let them try it for a while and see if it leads to success. This probably contradicts a lot of coaching laws because most coaches are control freaks who want to administrate as much of the athlete's life as possible. They feel like it's their job and, to some degree, it is.

However, the performances of lifters like Dimas, Martinez, Petrov, and Vardanian are evidence that individualization has value in our sport. As a coach, you will develop your own skills of analysis and intuition as your career goes on. If your experience leads you to think that an athlete is doing something wrong, then get in there and fix it. Trust your instincts. If your experience leads you to think that you just need to stop talking and let the athlete lift, then give it a try. Being a good coach doesn't mean you have to be constantly telling your athletes what to do. Sometimes, being a good coach means knowing when to keep quiet and let them figure it out for themselves. Are you going to make mistakes as you try to learn which one of these is called for? Absolutely. Why, did you think this was going to be easy?

STEINER

Matthias Steiner is a German weightlifter who won the Olympic gold medal in the +105 kilo weight class at the 2008 Olympics in Beijing. Steiner was not the favorite to win this meet. In fact, he had to attempt a clean and jerk of 258 kilos (568 pounds) for the victory. He had only one shot to make this lift, and it was almost twenty pounds more than he had ever lifted in his life. He made the lift and won the gold medal. It was one of the most amazing performances in weightlifting history. When he stood on the medal podium to receive his medal and listen to the German national anthem, he was holding a photo of his late wife Susann. She had been killed in a car accident the previous year, and he had decided to win the gold medal in honor of her memory. I wish the American media would have done more to publicize this story, because it's one of the best damn things I've ever heard in my life.

FUNKY LOCKOUT BLUES

When I was in my early twenties, I drove a 1981 Chevy Malibu station wagon. I bought it from my parents when I finished high school and drove it until I graduated from college and got my first full-time job. I loved this car, but it was one of the biggest pieces of crap in the galaxy. Every morning when I left my house to go to class, I would sit in the front seat of my car, put the key in the ignition, and pray to Valhalla that it would start. Sometimes it started, and sometimes it didn't. And if it didn't start, I had to combine some fast thinking and a kaleidoscope of foul language while I tried to get it running so I could make it to class on time. This probably happened seven or eight times a month... for six years. That's frustration, jack.

However, that wasn't the only frustrating pickle I ever had to grapple with. There have been others, obviously. And every one of you reading this article can think of your own predicaments from the past or the present where some common irritation keeps popping up. Your junker car, your annoying spouse, your lack of math skills, your toe fungus, whatever. The reason we're talking about this stuff is because there is probably nothing more frustrating for a weightlifter than not being able to complete the jerk after a successful clean. You've put in all the effort to clean the barbell, it's sitting on your shoulders, people have their cameras ready, the judge's finger is twitching on the white light button, and you crush the hopes of everybody in the room because you just can't find a way to stick it over your ears and complete the entire clean and jerk. All that effort in the clean was for nothing and now your mom is embarrassed because you're a lousy, disgusting jerker. For some athletes, this almost seems like an unconquerable nemesis. That's why this article is about jerking, plain and simple.

You need to know that I feel your pain, brothers and sisters. For the first few years of my weightlifting career, I was in this exact same swamp of failure. I had a fifteen kilo difference between what I could clean and what I could jerk, and I missed more jerks than I made in competition during this time. It was ridiculous. I knew how to perform the jerk, I was strong, my technique was solid, but the weight just wouldn't stay overhead when I was attempting my heaviest lifts. It was enough to make a grown man weep. If there would have been Jerk Prozac available, I would have had it loaded into a Pez dispenser.

This lasted until I was around twenty. And then I learned some things. I made some changes. I fixed a few problems that I had never thought of fixing because I didn't even know they were problems. By the time I was twenty-four, I was a legitimate jerking machine. I don't think I missed three jerks in competition for the next four or five years and I was lifting 30-40 kilos more than I had been in the younger years. So now, believe it or not, I'm going to hand you some of the solutions I discovered on a silver platter. You're about to become a better jerker as you sit where you are. You'd better be ready.

Make sure you're fishing in the right pond

First of all, this article is not going to be a technical analysis of how to perform the jerk. If you want that, then you need to buy Greg Everett's book, ask a coach to teach you, or watch some videos of Wes Barnett. All of those things will explain how to achieve technical magnificence in the jerk. Instead, we're going to look at some practical ideas to improve the jerking prowess of an athlete who already has a solid foundation of knowledge and technique.

One of the easiest steps in the jerking equation is to figure out if you're using the correct style. Are you going to be better at the push jerk, the squat jerk, or the split jerk? Right away, we need to make sure we're clear on the terminology. Split jerking is the most common jerk technique in weightlifting. This is the easily recognizable form where the athlete punches one foot forward and one foot backwards to lock the bar overhead in a sort of stride position. If you go to a weightlifting meet, the vast majority of the lifters you see will use the split jerk. The squat jerk, on the other hand, is a technique where the athlete punches under the bar by jumping the feet slightly out to the sides and descending into a deep squat. The bottom position of this jerk looks like a clean-grip snatch, and it has been popularized by some world-class lifters. Chinese Olympic Champion Zhan Xugang probably has the greatest squat jerk in history, and studying videos of his technique will give you a solid idea of what it's supposed to look like. Finally, the push jerk is a basically just a shallow version of the squat jerk. The feet are jumped into the squat position when punching under the bar, but the athlete does not descend into a full squat. Most push jerkers catch the weight in a position that looks like a half-squat. Some coaches refer to the push jerk as a "power jerk," which is fine. Greek legend Pyrros Dimas is one of the most famous push jerkers in history, although some of his biggest lifts drove him down deep enough into a position that was close to a squat jerk.

There is no rule written in stone that dictates which style of jerk an athlete should use. Whichever style gives the athlete the best results is the correct one for that particular individual. Most weightlifters in the world use the split jerk because it has historically yielded the highest marks. Most (not all) world records in the clean and jerk have been set with split jerks. However, this does not make it the universal rule for everyone. Some athletes are simply more comfortable with push jerking or squat jerking. Pyrros Dimas and his Greek teammate Kakhi Kakhiashvili both won three Olympic gold medals using push jerks. Dimas actually converted to the split jerk briefly in 1993 and the change simply did not work for him.

As a coach, my personal preference would be to teach the athlete how to perform the split jerk with the intention of using it exclusively. However, all weightlifters should also be taught how to perform the push jerk and it can be used as a terrific assistance exercise. If time passes by and the athlete has sustained difficulty with split jerking, it would be wise to give the push jerk a try. If the athlete learns the push jerk and quickly exceeds his/her best split jerk results, the coach may want to consider a full-time conversion. Obviously, this will need to be given attention on an individual case-by-case basis. The squat jerk will probably be a little trickier because of the extreme flexibility and strength it requires. The athletes will basically have to be able to perform a narrow grip overhead squat with the same weight as their top cleans. This requires a very special type of athlete with unique leverage.

Caveat! Caveat!

Although the idea of converting a split jerker into a push or squat jerker is always a viable option, a warning that needs to be mentioned is that the coach shouldn't rush to convert the athlete away from split jerks simply because the athlete is having difficulty. There are ways to fix a sloppy jerk without switching styles. As mentioned above, this article is not a tutorial on how to perform a jerk. However, it will examine some common mistakes and how to fix them. Here are a few of them:

Problem: The athlete is trying to jerk the bar with the upper body instead of using the power of the lower body. This is an easy one to spot. The next time an athlete has a bar on the shoulders and is preparing to jerk, take a look at the athlete's hands. If you can see that the athlete is gripping the bar tightly with the hands, it means he/she has already started to prepare for an arm-initiated movement. White knuckles, straining forearms, and purple fingers don't lie. If athletes attempt to jerk the bar overhead using the strength of the upper body, it will be a disaster. The arms and shoulders are simply not strong enough to lift a maximum clean weight over the head to a locked position. The power to complete the jerk has to come from the lower body.

Solution: Tell the athlete to loosen their hands before attempting the jerk. Some great jerkers even have the fingers slightly opened prior to the dip. Loosening the hands forces the athlete to use the legs. When I was getting started in weightlifting, I once heard a coach say that the drive of the legs should generate enough power to elevate the barbell to the level of the forehead, and that the arms shouldn't even be actively used until the bar is passing the scalp and the split has begun. This is an interesting way to describe the movement and just might be the proper verbal cue to give one of your athletes the correct mental perception of the lift.

Problem: The athlete is driving the bar forward when it comes off the shoulders and the lockout is not directly over the head. This could be caused by a variety of culprits. Therefore, multiple solutions are in order.

Solution: The athlete might be letting the elbows sag down during the dip phase. Watch the jerk from the side and see if the elbows are drooping when the athlete dips with the legs. If the elbows are drooping, then the shoulders are rounding forward as well. Both of these will cause the bar to be driven forward, away from the body, during the drive phase. A useful verbal cue for this problem is "big chest on the dip." When the athlete thinks about spreading the chest and maintaining a strong upright posture during the dip, the elbows are much less likely to sag because the position of the shoulder girdle will force them to stay up.

Solution: The athlete might have tight flexibility in the overhead position. Obviously, stretching is a necessary element to fixing this. However, jerks from behind the neck can be extremely beneficial in this situation. If you are unfamiliar with this exercise, it's exactly what it sounds like. The bar is placed on the back exactly like a back squat, and then the athlete simply performs the jerk. Because the starting position of the barbell is already behind the ears, the athlete has a much better chance of locking it out in the correct position over the head.

Solution: The athlete might be pushing the hips back (instead of straight down) during the dip phase. If the hips start to shift backwards during the dip, the resulting drive will be forward instead of straight up. Telling the athlete to "dip through the heels" is often helpful here. The athlete must mentally imagine the hips dropping straight down between the heels. Likewise, the athlete might also have his/her bodyweight on the front of the foot prior to the dip. This can result in the same forward problem. "Dip through the heels" will obviously communicate to the athlete that the weight should not be on the front of the foot before the jerk is initiated.

Problem: The athlete is having trouble locking out the bar on straight elbows overhead. This is clearly a technical problem and it is also one of the most common rule violations in the sport (pressout). Although there are some technique changes that can be made to fix a poor lockout, it must also be acknowledged that the problem could simply be a structural issue with the athlete's elbows. To state it clearly, some people just have really lousy elbow lockouts. The arms don't completely straighten and the athlete has all kinds of wobbly, bendy issues when the bar is overhead. These people will struggle with the Olympic lifts, period. However, let's make sure we understand that it is still possible to be a successful Olympic lifter even though the elbow lockout is shoddy. It's been done before.

Solution: Poor elbow lockout could be fixed by adjusting the width of the grip. The athlete's hands might need to be widened (or narrowed) to give the straight, snappy lockout we're looking for. This will obviously need to be considered in conjunction with the most beneficial grip for the clean, since the clean and jerk is a two-part movement. Poor lockout could also be caused by improper timing. If the athlete's feet are landing and planting on the platform too early, the elbows might still be fighting for lockout when the lower body has already fixed itself into position. Telling the athlete to synchronize the feet landing with the elbow lockout can give a proper sense of timing.

Some lifters will struggle with jerks their entire career. Stand behind an athlete sometime and look at their shoulders. You'll usually figure out which ones will be the best jerkers simply by seeing their physical structure. If the athlete has narrow, sloping shoulders, then jerking will be tough. The upper body is going to have to work extremely hard just to support the barbell during the dip phase because the shoulders naturally have a downward contour to them. Then, on the other hand, look at the athletes who have a square, wide look to their shoulders where the span from deltoid to deltoid looks like the top of a box. These will be the best jerkers because the barbell has a natural plateau to rest on while the dip and drive are taking place. Look at it this way; what would happen if you sat a fifty pound block of concrete on top of a cardboard toilet paper roll? The toilet paper roll would get crushed because it's just not a strong enough support base. Now, what if you took that same concrete block and sat it on top of a dictionary? That dictionary would have a much better chance to support the block because of its density and size. Likewise, an athlete with a wider, thicker support base for the barbell will probably have a stronger jerk than an athlete with a narrower, thinner base. This is why increased mass in the upper body often leads to greater results in the jerk.

There is nothing nicer than seeing an athlete absolutely stick a perfect jerk after a tough clean. American legend Jeff Michels was thrilling to watch because many of his best jerks were popped into lockout after tough, grinding, screaming cleans. Some people have a natural knack for it. And then there are the unlucky ones, who go to meets and clean massive weights easily only to have the jerk come crashing down on them like a fighter jet being shot down. Those are the ones who have to put in extra work, end of story. However, as a former pathetic jerker who went to jerk rehab and eventually developed into a jerking assassin, I can tell you that the struggle is worth it when you start getting those down signals. Happy jerking, amigos.

GIVE IT A LITTLE TUG: THE USE OF PULLS FOR WEIGHTLIFTERS

Don't you hate those times when you realize that you've forgotten to do something that was pretty important? This probably doesn't happen to most of you very often, because everybody knows that reading the Performance Menu sharpens your mind to the point where it could practically split the atom. But let's just assume that there are moments when you're in the middle of your busy life and then, all of a sudden, it occurs to you that you didn't do something that you really needed to take care of.

I think back to the wonderful, heartwarming days of my youth when my family would be driving in the station wagon on the way to a long road-trip vacation. Like clockwork, we would get six or seven miles down the road and either my mom, my brother, or I would realize that we forgot a toothbrush, swimming trunks, whatever. Aaahhh, the sentimental feelings I get when I recall my father's loving response to these little mistakes. "Good lord!! We're ten miles down the *!%&ing road now!! We're not turning around so you can go back and get your $#*!ing swimming trunks!!" It was like a Hallmark commercial… on crack.

The reason I'm bringing all of this up is that I recently realized that I have totally forgotten something pretty important over the last few years since I've been writing for this magazine. I've written articles on squats, jerks, several different technical aspects of the Olympic lifts, training programming, deadlifts, the whole ball of cheese. But when I looked in my computer file a few weeks ago where I keep all the Performance Menu articles I've done, it occurred to me that I've never written an article about the use of pulls. I'm talking about using snatch pulls and clean pulls in training to improve the performance of the snatch and clean.

I don't know what's going on, brothers and sisters. How could I have been writing for you all this time and never given you an article about one of the absolute most important components of a weightlifter's development? Pulls are essential if you want to snatch or clean bigger weights. I can't imagine trying to become a better weightlifter without using them. This is a truth that I believe in very strongly, but I understand that it's also a statement that not everybody agrees with. The use of pulls has been followed by a little controversy in the weightlifting circles, and we'll make sure we take a look at where this controversy comes from.

Mea culpa, guys. Good lord, I've never written an article about pulls, and you've been reading this &*%!ing magazine for years!! Better late than never, though. I'm going to jump right into the meat of this article without any more of my jazzy preamble banter. I don't want to waste any time, because pulls are just that important.

Let's get the basics out of the way…

Snatch or clean pulls are an assistance exercise for the development of the Olympic lifts. Most of you probably know what pulls are, but let's hit a quick explanation anyway. In a snatch or clean pull, the athlete basically performs the exact same movement as the snatch or clean. But when doing pulls, the movement stops at the top of the pull. There is no turnover or receiving position. Visualize a lifter doing a snatch or clean, and then hit pause with your brain when the lifter is at the fully extended top-pull position. The athlete is extended as tall as possible onto the toes with the shoulders shrugging, that's a completed pull. Conceptually, it's very similar to powerlifters using partial movements like deadlift lockouts in a power rack. The idea is that the lifters will perform pulls using weights that are heavier than their maximum snatches or cleans. In other words, a lifter who can snatch 200 pounds would use pulls in their workout by doing five sets of three repetitions with 215-225 pounds, somewhere in that area. The idea is that the pulling phase of the snatch or clean will be strengthened through overload. The 200-pound snatcher will build greater pulling strength by completing these movements with 225 pounds, which will allow the athlete to eventually snatch a personal record of 205 or 210 because the body has developed the power to handle this weight through multiple pull workouts.

It's important to mention that there is a difference between pulls and high pulls. When doing pulls, the arms stay straight throughout the entire movement. But when doing high pulls, the athlete extends into the finished pulling movement and also pulls the elbows upwards, bringing the bar up to the level of the chest. In other words, the arms pull up on the bar when doing high pulls, but they stay hanging straight when doing pulls.

Personally, I'm not a big fan of high pulls. I think the best way to incorporate pulls into a weightlifter's arsenal is to let the arms hang straight and focus on the movement of the legs, hips, back and shoulders. I don't think the movement of the high pull has a very close connection to what actually happens when a lifter performs a snatch or clean. There have been a few times in my career when I've seen elite-level lifters doing high pulls, but not often. The vast majority of the lifters I've seen or trained with over the years have preferred pulls.

Using straps when doing pulls is a general rule for weightlifters. Pulls are not a grip training exercise, and doing multiple sets and reps with a hook grip puts a serious beating on the thumbs, especially with the heavy weights that will be used for pulls. If the athlete uses straps, the focus can be put entirely on the pulling movement, which is why we're doing the damn things in the first place. For weight selection, many coaches like to use approximately 110% of the athlete's personal best in the competition lift. If the lifter can snatch 150 kilos, then multiplying 150x1.1 gives us 165 kilos, which is a good weight for that particular athlete to use for pulls. Some coaches get aggressive with pulls and decide to really load the weights up. I've seen athletes who clean 90 kilos using 145 for their pulls, which brings us to one of the most important issues in this discussion.

The technique of the pull must duplicate the movement of the athlete's competition lifts. You heard me. Your clean pulls should basically look exactly like your cleans, just without the turnover and completion. If you decide to use clean pulls in your workouts and you load the weights up drastically above 110% of your clean, there is a strong chance that there are going to be some technical flaws in your pulls. The back will likely not stay perfectly tight and flat, speed will be compromised, the butt might rise too quickly when pulling from the floor, etc. When you get to this point, you are simply practicing incorrect movements. There is no point to doing pulls if using them is going to strengthen technical flaws. Sure, it's great to be able to load all those bumpers on the bar and impress everybody in your gym. But the translation of your pulling strength into your actual snatch or clean will be very minimal. The speed of your pulls should be as close as possible to the speed of your full lifts. It isn't realistic to expect to move 110% of your best snatch with exactly the same speed as your snatches, but they should be in the same ballpark. If those snatch pulls start to look more like deadlifts than snatches, you need to strip some weight off the bar.

The world according to Jaber…

My personal belief is that pulls should be finished with the athlete extending as high up on the toes as possible. However, this idea comes from my basic philosophy on how to perform the Olympic lifts. I have always believed that optimum weightlifting technique requires the athlete to stretch the body as tall as possible in the finish of the pull. The lifter should be pushing up onto the toes, the hips should be totally extended, and the shoulders should be shrugging violently upwards. That's just how I think it should be done, folks.

However, it's important to mention at this point that there are some voices in the weightlifting world that have different opinions. I just read an article on the internet a few weeks ago where the writer said the athlete should perform the entire pulling movement with the weight on the heels of the foot. I totally disagree with this idea. I have always taught athletes to feel their bodyweight in the middle of their foot until the final extension of the pull, when the goal is to drive up onto the toes before jumping the feet outwards into the receiving position.

As I said, there are coaches who teach things differently. When I was brainstorming this article, I looked around on YouTube to find some clips of athletes performing snatch or clean pulls, hoping I could include the video links here. But I couldn't find one freaking video where anybody was doing their pulls correctly. Admittedly, most of the videos I looked at were not elite weightlifters. That probably explains a lot. However, I did watch some old video of the 2001 World Weightlifting Championships right before I started writing this piece, and I got to see superheavyweight world champion Jaber Salem from Qatar snatching 210 kilos (462 pounds). Jaber's technique is a great visual demonstration of what I'm describing. Because he was raised in the Bulgarian system (he's actually Yanni Marchakov from Bulgaria, but Qatar offered him a big chunk of cash to lift for their country), Jaber gets incredible extension into the top of his pull, rising up onto the toes before jumping his feet out with a stomp as he catches the bar overhead. Almost all of the great Bulgarian lifters have similar technique, including 77 kilo world champion Zlatan Vanev, who is one of the best technicians I've ever seen. It's not just a Bulgarian thing, though. The Russian superheavyweight who finished second behind Jaber with a 451 pound snatch executed his lifts in the same manner. The only thing about Jaber's technique I don't like is that he jumps forward slightly, which is generally a major no-no in weightlifting. But he snatches 462 pounds. I guess he can jump wherever he wants.

There will be people who point at great lifters like Pyrros Dimas of Greece and mention that Dimas basically stayed flat-footed throughout his pulling movement, which is different from what I just said about proper weightlifting technique. It's true, Dimas did pull almost entirely flat-footed. And that point brings us to a weightlifting truth that many coaches just can't seem to understand. There is more than one way to lift big weights. No technical model is universal, and no technique philosophy is dogma. World records have been lifted by people who extend onto the toes and jump the feet out with a stomp, and world records have been lifted by people who keep most of their foot on the floor for most of the lift. I have always believed that if you watch enough world championship footage, the majority of the great lifters you see will lift with technique that is closer to Jaber's, the extend-on-the-toes-and-jump-outward model that I described. There's a lot of evidence out there to back this up, and that's why I teach weightlifting the way I do. But I would never say that there's only one way to perfect these movements.

Long story short, I think pulls should finish with extension onto the toes at the top. If you want to do pulls with your heels on the floor, knock yourself out.

Other incredibly important and intensely critical issues…

Let's do a rapid fire list of other ideas regarding pulls:

Pulls can be performed from the floor, from the hang, from blocks, etc. I personally like doing all pulls from the floor because I think that relates most closely with the movements that will take place on a competition platform. But a little variety never hurt anybody, and doing pulls from different positions can be a great way to mix things up for the athlete.

Sets of three-five are good repetitions for pulls, hitting three-five sets right after the competition lifts have been finished in training. In other words, after you've finished your snatches, do five sets of three in snatch pulls with around 110% of your highest snatch (then, do your squats). That's a solid plan, but remember that the 110% number isn't etched in stone anywhere. My coach used to have us occasionally do three sets of five reps with 100%. Five reps of pulls with your clean max will give those spinal erectors a good test. Doing pulls two or three times a week is good planning, and eliminating them fourteen days before a competition is even better planning.

As I said, pulls should be an essential component of the weightlifter's preparation. I would never train anybody who was serious about lifting without including pulls. I've heard some coaches say over the years that they don't think pulls are important because they believe in "the Bulgarian training model" and the Bulgarians don't do them. Okay, let me say a couple of things about that. First of all, the Bulgarians do pulls. I've seen them. It might be true that they don't use pulls as one of the primary exercises with their top lifters, but they do include them in different phases of their preparation. If people tell you differently, remind them that much of the information we've received in America about the Bulgarian approach has been skewed. And even if the Bulgarians don't do a lot of pulls... so what? The Russians do pulls in their training, and they've been cranking out the best lifters in the world for fifty years. So stick that in your pudding and stir it.

They make your core stronger. They make your technique better. They make your glutes and traps harder, which is going to increase the love and respect you get from the weightlifting community. I mean seriously people...there are just too many freaking positives to walk away from when it comes to pulls.

I've met some lifters who say they don't like doing pulls. Okay, fine. Do you like getting the crap kicked out of you by other weightlifters? No? Then do your pulls. You can mix up the sets and reps, mix up the weights, mix up the starting position you do them from, etc. You can even mix up when you do them in your workout, although I would always do them before squats.

So there you have it people, an article about one of the most fundamental weightlifting tools that it took me three years to think of. Maybe I'll put together some more keen articles in the next few months about topics like why it's important not to stab yourself, how drinking bleach is a bad idea, stuff like that. Now that the most obvious things in the world have made their way to the front of my brain, the possibilities are endless.

BONES OF IRON

SECTION TWO:
COMPETITIVE EXPERIENCE

Combining Olympic weightlifting and powerlifting, I've competed in over one hundred meets in my career. Many of you are either competitive strength athletes or you're at least thinking about becoming one. First of all, I highly recommend taking the plunge and doing this if you know how to perform the lifts to competition rules standards. The worst thing that could happen is you lose $30 on an entry fee, you have a bad experience, and you decide it's not for you. The best thing that could happen is you find a new passion in your life.

I've been very fortunate because I've trained with some of the greatest weightlifting athletes and coaches in the world. Even though I went to college and graduate school for my professional career, my weightlifting education came from the School of Hard Knocks. The things I've learned about training, life, and myself have been immeasurable. Here are a few of my favorite ones.

LESSONS FROM ROMANIA

Nicu Vlad is one of the greatest weightlifters of all time. The Romanian legend won the Olympic gold medal at the 1984 Los Angeles games when he was only twenty-one years old, and that was only the beginning of his amazing career. Vlad went on to win the silver medal at the 1988 Olympics, the bronze at the 1996 Olympics (when he was thirty-three), and three world championships in 1984, 1986, and 1990. However, the accomplishment that Vlad is probably most famous for is his all-time world record snatch of 200.5 kilos in the old 100 kilo bodyweight class. He is the heaviest lifter in history to snatch double bodyweight, and many weightlifting experts believe that Vlad is one of the most technically perfect weightlifters of all time. His snatch technique has been the learning model for thousands of young weightlifters over the last two decades. So you can imagine how I felt when I found out that I was going to have the opportunity to train with Vlad for three weeks at the Olympic Training Center in Colorado Springs during the summer of 1990.

Nicu and his coach, Dragomir Cioroslan, came to the United States in 1990 to spend the summer training at various locations around the country. They spent most of this visit in Colorado Springs, and the national junior squad training camp was held at the OTC during the same time. I was invited to train at this camp, which meant that I was going to be working out in the same gym with an athlete whose pictures I had taped up on the walls of the gym where I worked out at home. I was seventeen years old and Nicu Vlad had been my weightlifting idol long before I knew he was coming to the United States. This was literally the opportunity of a lifetime, and this article will examine just a fraction of the many lessons I learned during that memorable summer.

First, the formal details of training...

I recall meeting Dragomir and Nicu for the first time. Dragomir, who was one of the friendliest people I had ever met in my life, smiled broadly and shook my hand with gusto as he looked me in the eye and exclaimed, "My name is Dragomir, how are you?!" After that, I was introduced to the big man, who shook my hand with his thick paw and growled, "Nicu Vlad," as he glanced at me with the same interest he probably showed in his morning bowel movement. Nicu was polite and respectful, but he had a quiet intensity in his personality that was obvious. This man was a legend, and everybody knew it. You gave him a wide berth.

Nicu usually trained twice a day, and his workouts were broken up into short segments. He generally performed the classic lifts along with front squats, back squats, and RDLs (more on that later). I never saw him spend any time doing supplemental exercises such as push presses, overhead squats, etc. He often performed his squats in the mornings and his competition lifts in the afternoons. In a typical afternoon session, he would train one of the competition lifts (snatch or clean and jerk) for around thirty minutes and then go outside the gym to lie down in the grass and relax for a while. After twenty or thirty minutes, he would come back in the gym to train again, often hitting the other competition lift. After this second session, he would sometimes go back outside to take another relaxation break before the next segment or sometimes he would go straight into a squatting or pulling movement, depending on which lifts he had trained that morning. Basically, Dragomir had him on a European-style program that combined many of the Russian and Bulgarian principles that we have all studied over the years. He was training around seven to nine times per week, with the morning sessions usually taking place around ten o'clock and the afternoon sessions around three or four. It's important to note that Nicu was twenty-seven years old during this time, which is generally considered a little old for most hardcore European training systems. I believe his volume and exercise selection had been narrowed to accommodate his age.

Nicu was training to compete at the 1990 Goodwill Games in Washington at the end of the summer, so I was able to see him train when he was around six weeks out from a meet. The top lifts I saw him perform in training during this time are as follows: 185 snatch, 210 clean and jerk (he clean and jerked 210, brought the weight down to his shoulders, and jerked it a second time). Nicu's all-time best official lifts are 200.5 in the snatch and 237.5 in the clean and jerk. But those lifts had been done in 1986; during the 1990 time period when I saw him, he was usually hitting around 190/220 in meets. Therefore, 185 and 210 were working pretty close to his top results at the time. In the supplemental lifts, I saw multiple sets of three in the back squats with 250-260, and RDL sets of three usually performed with 250-260. The squats and RDLs with 260 were, as far as the eye could tell, practically effortless. He did not squat with any of the massive weights that many Americans *think* the top European lifters handle on a daily basis. Also, the jerk was his weak spot and, because of this, he almost always lowered the weight to his shoulders and performed two reps of the jerk for every clean.

But despite the amazing work capacity and kilograms Nicu was capable of handling, the most phenomenal aspect of his training was definitely his technique. When I first became an Olympic weightlifter, a great coach told me that one of the elements of having perfect technique meant you could "make 50 kilos look exactly the same as 150 kilos." Vlad was the best example of this rule that I have ever seen in my career. Every movement of his body from his back position to his foot placement to his acceleration in the second pull was identical, regardless of the weight on the bar. When he performed snatches and cleans, he would usually power snatch or power clean the light weights, catching them in a high receiving position. And, as the weight got progressively heavier, he would simply catch the bar gradually lower and lower until he was hitting his top weights and catching them near rock-bottom. Nicu jumped his feet forcefully off the platform when he was extending the second pull and going under the bar, producing a loud *slap!* when his feet hit the platform as he turned his wrists over and caught the weight. Not every great lifter has utilized the same "feet jumping" technique as Vlad, obviously. There are some great lifters who simply lift their feet just high enough to slide them out and re-position them as they receive the bar. But Vlad's technique involved violent jumping of the feet and many lifters, including myself, formed their own technique from emulating him. Everything about his movements was a textbook combination of speed, tightness, precision, and strength. Any weight-lifter who wants to be successful would be wise to study the technique of Nicu Vlad, as we all did during our summer of watching him train.

A quick 185 snatch, then some RDLs...

One afternoon, many of the junior squad lifters were in the OTC game room playing pool and PacMan when Wes Barnett stuck his head in the door and told everybody, "Vlad's going heavy in his workout." We all ran out of the game room, across the hockey field, and down the hill to the gym so we could see some big weights. Nicu was warming up in the snatch at the time, and we all quietly took seats around the gym to watch the big show. After his normal warm up, snatching 70, 90, 110, 130, 140, 150, and 160 with ease, he put 170 on the bar. We were all shocked to see him miss the 170, but then he repeated the weight a few minutes later and made it easily. He jumped to 175 and missed the weight behind him twice, and then jumped to 180 and missed that weight twice as well. Most of us were wondering what in the hell was going on, as he was clearly in good shape and strong enough to make these weights. I will never forget what he did next.

He loaded 185 on the bar. This time, as he stood in front of the bar preparing for the lift, he stood motionless, tilted his head back and closed his eyes in the famous Vlad-concentration pose we had all seen him strike on the platform at the Olympics and world championships. He had not done this before any of the other lifts of his workout, and the gym went completely silent. After ten seconds, he reached down, grabbed the bar, and nailed the easiest, strongest snatch of the day.

I learned a lot about mental discipline as I watched this workout. After his missed snatch attempts, Nicu had no reaction whatsoever. He did not get visibly upset or discouraged in any way. His face remained stoic and he simply progressed to the next weight, confident that he would make any technical corrections that were needed. When he got to 185, which I later learned was the weight he had planned to hit that day, he just applied an extra level of concentration and focus.

It was a big weight, he was having a bad workout, and he needed to tap into his extra reservoir of inner strength, mojo, or whatever you want to call it. Because he was a world champion, his mojo did not involve jumping around like a crackhead, punching himself in the face, or kicking the bar. His fire burned *inside*, and it burned hot. And after he made the 185, he simply went on with the rest of his workout. No celebration, actions of deep relief, or pissing and moaning because he hadn't had a perfect workout. It was all just a day at the office for Nicu Vlad.

Then he started performing an exercise we saw him do regularly. It looked a lot like a stiff-legged deadlift, only he bent his knees slightly and displaced his hips backwards as he lowered the bar. He would regularly do this exercise with 250 kilos or more, and he even did a personal record set of 300x3 at the end of the camp. Somebody in the gym asked Nicu and Dragomir what the exercise was called. They said that they did not have a special name for it, and so one of the American lifters suggested that it could be called a "Romanian Deadlift" or RDL. Now, here we are eighteen years later, and this exercise has become a common staple in workout routines all across this country. I've always considered it a privilege that I was present when the RDL was officially named.

The Nicu Vlad Charm School…

Vlad was a fairly quiet, reserved personality, probably due mostly to the fact that his English at the time was relatively limited. With the English that he was able to speak, he was always happy to engage in conversation and joke around. I recall one night in the OTC dorm when a tall swimmer was walking down the hall and accidentally bumped into Nicu, knocking him back a step. The swimmer apparently thought he was a tough guy, because he just glanced around and kept walking without excusing himself. Wes Barnett jokingly told Nicu to go give the guy a beating. Nicu looked at Wes and shook his head saying "What?" because he didn't understand. Wes pointed at the swimmer and punched his fist into his palm five or six times. Nicu understood, but he stopped Wes and said, "No." Then he punched his own fist into his palm one time, looked at Wes and said, "Just one." He was telling us that he could knock the guy out with one shot!

Nicu also gave out a piece of advice that I now realize is probably the greatest lesson I've ever learned in weightlifting and life in general. This particular junior squad camp had several young athletes who would later go on to become great American lifters in the 1990s. Names like Barnett, Gough, McRae, Patao, and my dorm roommate Pete Kelley were all there. These individuals were hardworking, driven, competitive animals who were hungry to move up in the national rankings. However, there were also several young athletes who had made the junior squad and earned their way to the camp, but showed some of the worst attitudes I have seen in my years as an athlete. These were spoiled brats who whined constantly about the gym being too small, the bars not spinning well enough, the dorms being too hot, the taste of the dining hall food, and every other free benefit that had been given to them. They did not train hard, complained incessantly, back-talked the coaches and OTC staff, and threw temper tantrums in the gym when they missed lifts. Not surprisingly, almost all of them quit the sport within the next few years.

Nicu and Dragomir used to watch these kids silently and shake their heads in disgust. It was obvious what they were thinking. Then, USA Weightlifting magazine decided to do an interview with Vlad, so Dragomir acted as his interpreter to answer their questions. At one point, the reporter asked Nicu what he thought about training with our top young junior lifters. Although I'm not quoting him word-for-word, I remember his answer clearly and it was this: "In Romania, I train on a bar that is bent. My gym has bad lighting and very little heat in the winters. Here in America, you have everything you need to train. It's not in the bar or the gym or the platform… it's in you."

The message, which I consider almost a biblical principle, is that the strength you possess in your heart will be the deciding element in your weightlifting career. Adversity is the name of the game in this sport, and the only factor that can propel an athlete to success is sheer force of will. Physical talent is not enough. There are armies of physically talented athletes out there. The ones like Nicu Vlad, who refuse to allow anything to defeat them, will be the last ones standing. This attitude drove Nicu forward to victory at the World Championship that same year, and then eventually to the 1996 Olympics in Atlanta, where, at the age of thirty-three, he snatched 197.5 in the 108 class, winning the third Olympic medal of his illustrious career.

I could write an entire book about all the other things I saw, heard, and learned during those weeks. Vlad told us that Yuri Zacharevich from the Soviet Union had rack jerked 300 kilos in training. Vlad told us that Naim Suleymanoglu owned eight houses in Turkey. Vlad told us that we were all idiots for spending our recovery time having chicken fights in the OTC pool instead of resting for our next workout. During his trip, somebody printed up some "Nicu Vlad Summer US Tour 1990" tank tops and sold them. I bought one and wore it as religiously as the stoners at my high school wore their Megadeth t-shirts. It was an exciting summer that marked the beginning of some great US lifting careers. I was lucky to be there. We all were.

BORN AGAIN...
FOR THE FIRST TIME

Not long ago, I spent some time reading posts on the Catalyst Athletics Weight-lifting and Powerlifting forum. Aside from the fact that I like reading about weightlifting practically all the time, I thought the forums would give me a little insight into what our Performance Menu readers are talking about these days and, from there, I might get some ideas for future articles. It's all part of this new plan of mine to be more considerate of the feelings of other people.

Interestingly, there were several posts from individuals who are about to take the plunge and compete in their first Olympic Weightlifting competition. It was fun to read about the nervousness, uncertainty, and excitement that comes along with the idea of walking out on a competition platform in front of a bunch of people for the first time. They say that one of the average human being's greatest fears is public speaking. Standing up in front of a group of people and talking... that's enough to send most people into a hammerhead panic that could end with involuntary bladder discharge. Knowing this, we can assume that the idea of standing in front of a group of people in a tight spandex outfit and trying to lift heavy weights overhead without wiping out is probably even more threatening and scary.

So if there is so much fear and risk involved, why do people want to walk on that platform and compete? Everyone has his own answer. Some people are looking for a purpose in their life. Some people simply enjoy thrills. Many people like the idea of testing themselves and finding out just how strongly they stack up against others who practice their same discipline. And almost everybody likes to try something fun. I started lifting in weightlifting competitions almost twenty years ago and I've lifted in almost one hundred meets. And after all this time, my first competition is still as fresh in my memory as if it happened yesterday. I know now that the moment when I grabbed a barbell, snatched it, and waited for the down signal for the first time was one of the most important moments of my life. Everything about me was changed after my first meet. Weightlifting became, and continues to be, a spiritual pursuit. It's my religion. Throughout our sport's history, hundreds of athletes have experienced the same life change after their first meet as well. Our sport offers almost no money and promises pain, so only fanatics will survive for the long haul. The first competition, in many cases, is the moment of conception for these fanatics.

Because we all know that anything worth doing is worth doing right, it should be useful to discuss competitive weightlifting and how to prepare for your first meet... as well as your third and your fourth and your seventy-fifth. Now, some of you might be reading this article and saying to yourself, "I'm a Crossfitter and have no interest in competitive lifting, so thanks for wasting my time this month, Foremong." Hold your horses. I'm willing to bet my last peso we can find some useful tips in here for anybody who exercises in any gym for any reason, so let's organize our thoughts into one of my favorites... a top-three list.

This Month's Top Three Tips for Competitive Weightlifters

1. Don't focus on winning your first competition

If you are lucky, you will get spanked by an experienced, national-level lifter when you compete in your first meet. That's not a typo... you read that correctly. You should hope and pray that one of our country's top studs shows up to compete in the first meet you lift in. In my opinion, the best thing that can happen to a rookie is to have his/her eyes opened wide by a hardcore elite lifter who can lift weights you can't even dream of yet. If you have the right kind of personality to be a weightlifter (or just a human being who wants to be successful), you will have a ten-thousand degree fire in your belly after you see this animal hitting huge attempts on that platform. It should be a moment of inspiration, not demoralization.

We live in a me-generation, I-want-to-be-successful-in-everything-right-away-without-working-for-it culture, and this causes many people to run away from pursuits that will take months and years to perfect. Maybe this is part of the reason why weightlifting is a shrinking sport in our country. Who knows for sure? The only thing that is certain is that even genetically gifted athletes like Wes Barnett and Tara Nott had to spend lots and lots of time training before they made it to the top of the rock pile. And along the way, they had moments when they were thumped in competition. If you happen to compete against a Wes or Tara in your first meet, you will get thumped. And you should walk away from the competition chomping at the bit to get back in the gym and start making progress so that, one day, you will be the one at the meet that all the young bucks look up to. Getting beaten in your first meet should not be a shameful experience. It should make you hungry.

In my first meet, I competed in the old 90 kilo class. I was seventeen years old, had only been training for a few months prior to the meet, and I had never been coached by anybody. My technique was disgusting, and I only totaled 180 kilos (80 kilo snatch and 100 kilo clean and jerk). The other lifter competing in the 90 kilo class against me snatched 130 and clean and jerked 165 for a 295 total. He was four years older than me and he had been training for five or six years, and his lifting left quite a dent in my brain. I watched every move this cat made. I watched how he warmed up, how he acted between attempts, how he chalked his hands, how he taped his thumbs, how he stood over the bar and visualized the attempt before he reached down to grab it, everything. His performance stayed in my memory for a long time as my weightlifting journey began.

It took me three years to reach that 295 total I saw in my first meet. Those three years were amazingly tough and I loved every minute of them. And when I finally hit this 295 total in a meet, I'm positive that there were some greenhorns lifting in their first meet who probably thought a 295 total seemed as immoveable as Stonehenge. I can only hope that weightlifting's version of the Circle of Life took place there and some of these greenhorns decided to commit to breaking through their own walls, just as I did after I got owned at my first meet.

2. Train with short rest periods

The biggest loop I was thrown for when I came to my first weightlifting meet was how the actual competition was run. Through my prior experience of competing in powerlifting, I had known about the "rounds system." This is a system where the competition goes through a first attempt round, then a second attempt round, and then a third attempt round. In other words, every athlete does their first attempts, then they all do their second attempts, etc. Every powerlifting meet I have ever attended has used this system. However, Olympic Lifting uses a progressive-bar system, where the weight on the bar continues to move up and the athletes simply take their attempts when their individual weights are on the bar. The biggest difference between these two systems is how much time the lifter will have between attempts. In powerlifting, the length of time stays approximately the same between each attempt. In weightlifting, the time varies. The athlete might have ten minutes between attempts if he/she is taking large jumps (10-15 kilos), or there might only be two minutes between attempts if the athlete has to repeat an attempt.

Because of this, athletes should always make an effort to prepare for the worst case scenario. This means you should condition yourself in such a way that you can take heavy attempts successfully with only two or three minutes of rest. Over the years, I've worked with a lot of athletes who like to take huge breaks between heavy attempts in the gym. They'll chalk up, snatch a heavy weight, and then sit down and rest for eight minutes before chalking up for the next one. If you train like this, not only is it going to drag out your workouts for hours, it's also going to put you in a tight spot if you go to a weightlifting meet and you have to follow yourself between each of your attempts. You could easily be called to take your first, second, and third attempts in a total span of seven minutes. Knowing this, you'll be in a major pickle if your physiology isn't adapted to these short rest intervals.

The easiest way to escape this trap is simply to look at the clock in your gym and only allow yourself a couple of minutes between each set. It might take some getting used to, especially if you've previously trained yourself to sit on a bench like a garden slug for ten minutes between sets. But the rewards in competition will be massive. You'll never run out of gas if you have to take max attempts back-to-back, and a six-minute rest break will feel like paradise if you happen to get one.

3. Train with distractions

Let's use a little hypothetical situation to examine this one, shall we? Imagine your own gym, where you train every day. For the sake of this situation, we'll say you have six platforms, six Eleiko bars, and plenty of weights in your gym. Now, there are several athletes who train with you on a regular basis but I want to specifically look at two of them... a female lifter named Cindy Doodlekicker and a male lifter named Bob Rammer. Cindy and Bob aren't related or dating or anything. They're just lifters who train in your gym. However, Cindy and Bob are both extremely particular about their training routines. Cindy has a platform in the gym that she identifies as "her platform." She trains on this platform every day; it's her special little place. If anybody in the gym shows up earlier than her and starts training on her platform, Cindy gets upset because her routine is being disrupted. On top of that, Cindy is a little spitfire who has no problem getting in somebody's face and letting them know that they're training on "her platform." Everybody in the gym knows how Cindy is, so they just play along and let her have her platform all to herself so she doesn't have a panic attack.

Then, we have Bob. Bob has a platform he considers "his platform," just like Cindy, but Bob takes it a step further and has a specific bar he likes to train on. There is nothing different about this bar. It has the same spin, grip, etc. as every other bar in the gym. But Bob has had some good workouts on this bar and so he absolutely has to use it every day. If somebody else is working out on his bar when he gets to the gym, Bob will insist that he gets to share that bar with the other lifter. They can just change the weights to accommodate each of them on every set. It doesn't matter that the other lifter can snatch 170 and Bob snatches 82. Bob has to use his bar, so everybody has to be understanding.

Most of us know the types of people we're talking about. These are control freaks who have to have the entire gym environment exactly the way they want it when they train. Often, it doesn't just stop with the platforms or the bars. I've trained with lifters who throw fits over the radio station that's playing, the conversations taking place around them, the room temperature, and the amount of chalk that gets peppered around the floor. Now, make sure you understand that there is nothing wrong with having a favorite bar or platform. Most lifters do. But there is definitely something wrong with getting bent out of shape if you don't get to train on your favorite bar or platform.

Here are a few of the problems with behavior like this. First of all, everybody in the gym probably hates Cindy and Bob. They all play nice because they know they have to work out together, but there is still an unspoken agreement in the gym that everybody hates Bob's guts and wishes he and Cindy would quit the sport, find another gym, or die. Second, you can't train like this if you're planning to be a competitive weightlifter because weightlifting competitions throw you completely out of your control environment. Unfamiliar bars, unfamiliar surroundings, unfamiliar people. Every distraction and irritation you can imagine will pop up in a meet at some point if you compete long enough. People will walk right in front of you while you're hitting a big warm-up snatch. Babies will cry in the audience while you're attempting a personal record. Competition venues will sometimes be much hotter or colder than you're used to. Dozens of little unexpected irritations will spring up at weightlifting meets, so do yourself a favor and train in a way that allows you to lift successfully regardless of any of them. When I competed at the 2004 Olympic Trials, the sound system was blaring the song "She Bangs" by William Hung while I was warming up. We couldn't even get the Ricky Martin version, apparently. Try getting to the biggest competition of your life and having to block out the wailing of a snaggletooth American Idol reject as you prepare to compete. Do yourself a favor and lock in your mind on the barbell, any barbell, when you go to the gym every day. Let everything else roll off your back.

Actually, let's finish with tip #3 ½...
Because of our commitment to customer service at the Performance Menu, we'll throw in one more tittle of advice for aspiring weightlifters. I suppose the nicest way to put this is to say that you will encounter some... personalities when you go to weightlifting meets. What do I mean?

When I went to my first meet, I weighed in and then went to sit in the warm-up room and wait for the action to start. Other lifters were starting to mill around, and it was obvious that most of them knew each other. They shook hands, guy-hugged, chatted about how training had been going, etc. It was also obvious that none of them knew me. But after a few minutes, an older lifter approached me. He looked like he was around thirty years old and he had some muscle on him, but his hair was going in nine different directions and one of his eyeballs wouldn't stop twitching. I don't know who he had talked to about me, but he knew I had previously been a powerlifter. I have a very good memory when it comes to lifting, so I can get pretty close to a word-for-word recitation of my conversation with this gentleman. I'll just call him "Harry" to protect his identity.

Harry: "Hi, how's it going?"
Me: "Good, how are you?"
Harry: "Pretty good. Hey, I heard from somebody that you compete in powerlifting."
Me: "Yeah, I do."
Harry: "That's cool. I'd like to compete in powerlifting too. I think it would be fun."
Me: "Yeah, it's a lot of fun. You should do it."
Harry: "Do they do drug testing in powerlifting?"

Me: "Yeah, they do drug testing."
Harry: "They test you for steroids, right?"
Me: "Yeah, they test you for steroids."
Harry: "So coke and speed are okay?"
Me: (pause) "Huh?"
Harry: "You can do stuff like coke, speed, you know? That stuff is okay?"
Me: "Uuuhhh, I think they test for that stuff too."
Harry: "Really?"
Me: "Yeah, really."
Harry: "Okay, thanks for the heads up. Are you a Christian?"
Me: "A Christian?"
Harry: "Yeah, a born-again Christian?"
Me: "I guess so."
Harry: "Cool. Me too. Have a good meet today!"
Me: "Yeah... you too."

End of conversation, true story.

There should be a lot of great camaraderie at the weightlifting meets you attend. One of the best parts of being a weightlifter is the friendships and bonds you develop with people. You all choose to spend a huge part of your life in a common endeavor. You understand the same frustrations and rewards of your sport. Because of this, you tend to meet a lot of people who are a lot like you. But as with any culture, you will run into the occasional whack-job. Don't be surprised if you encounter a little dysfunctional behavior when you come to your first competition.

Fortunately, one of the things you find out quickly in this sport is that almost everyone is willing to help out the newbies. Weightlifters love weightlifters. When a new lifter pops up on the scene, most experienced coaches and athletes will be enthusiastic and supportive. This is a tribal sport, and new members are always welcome. Because of this, first-meet lifters who have been flying solo shouldn't feel any hesitation or apprehension about asking for help. If it's possible for you to get three steps ahead of the game and make arrangements to have a coach who will work with you at your first meet, you'll eliminate a lot of headaches. And if you take the time to cover all the other bases we've mentioned, you might be on the way to a terrific experience that will drive some new goals into your brain like thumbtacks. You might stumble onto your lifetime sport. You might even go on to conquer some of the other fears in your life after you've competed on the platform... like public speaking. After all, stranger things have happened.

HEALTH

My coach, John Thrush, got to have dinner with Bob Hoffman once. Bob Hoffman, for those who don't know, is referred to as the Father of World Weightlifting. He basically built the sport of weightlifting starting in the 1930s, along with inventing protein powder, nutrition bars, and the culture of physical fitness and health. John had dinner with him at a meet when Hoffman was older and already established as a god in the world of strength sports. John ordered a cheeseburger and fries and when the waiter brought the food, Hoffman told John, "You shouldn't eat those fries. They're unhealthy." John was in awe of Hoffman, so he didn't touch them. Hoffman started a lecture about the importance of health and nutrition. As he continued speaking, he started reaching over to John's plate and eating his fries. After a half an hour, Hoffman had delivered a lecture on the virtue of healthy eating while simultaneously eating every one of John's fries. God bless him.

BANANAS, CHOCOLATES, AND A BIG RUSSIAN BEAR

Academy Award-winning actor Tom Hanks was giving an interview once and he was describing a job he had early in his career, before he was a big name, where he had worked with a group of actors and directors who were much more experienced and skilled than he was. It was a tough situation, as he described it, because he was working in a talent pool that was way over his head. However, instead of whining and complaining when he remembered it all, he spoke of the whole thing as a valuable time that made him much better as an actor and a professional. One of the quotes he used during this interview was, "You never learn anything unless you get your butt kicked first." This line always stuck with me and I've come to believe that Hanks was right, in a lot of ways. In application to weightlifting and professional life, I think one of the best moves you can ever make is to surround yourself with people who are better than you. You're forced to work twice as hard and learn twice as fast if you want to move up and become an equal to these people, instead of staying at the bottom of the totem pole and accepting your role as the wanna-be. Obviously, being around people who are better than you is going to put you in a position where you feel defeat and inferiority at times. But that defeat should sharpen your hunger and, hopefully, the end result will be that you found a way to step up your game and compete on an even level with the top players. These ideas are exactly what I think about when I remember a moment in 2000 when I got a chance to compete against the best weightlifter on the planet.

Andrei Chemerkin won the Olympic gold medal in the 1996 Atlanta games. A massive twenty-four-year-old Russian superheavyweight, Andrei pulled out one of the greatest clutch lifts in weightlifting memory when he crushed a 260 kilo clean and jerk (a weight he had never made before) on his last attempt to defeat Germany's Ronny Weller and take the gold medal. It was an amazing moment that concluded one of the greatest superheavyweight competitions in Olympic history. After it was over, Andrei went on to establish himself as an almost unbeatable figure during the next four years. He followed up his Olympic victory with the 1997 World Championship, where he duplicated his Olympic final-attempt heroics by clean and jerking 262.5 kilos to once again beat Ronny Weller. Two more world championship titles in 1998 and 1999 gave Chemerkin an aura of invincibility. Not only was he the strongest weightlifter walking god's green earth, he was also the consummate pressure performer. The big man proved several times that he possessed one of the most important qualities an athlete can have… the ability to put up his greatest performances when his back was against the wall and he only had one shot left. Many people, myself included, began to regard Andrei in the same fashion as Alexeev during his prime. He was the king, plain and simple.

Knowing this, I knew it would be one of the highlights of my career when I found out that I was going to compete against Chemerkin at the 2000 World University Championships in Montreal. I qualified to compete for the US team in the superheavyweight class, and it had been widely advertised that Andrei was going to lift at this meet. I never knew exactly why he chose to travel all the way to Canada for this competition. The meet was held in June, only a few months before the Sydney Olympics, where he was obviously going to be attempting to defend his title. Although there were several outstanding international athletes at this university worlds, no superheavyweights were in attendance that had any chance to compete with the big man. But regardless of any reasons or details, the strongest weightlifter in the universe was planning to show up at this meet and I was going to lift on the same platform. I saw some amazing things on this trip and I learned some of the best lessons of my life. Here's how it went…

Montreal…

When I arrived in Montreal for the competition, the buzz was working overtime. Everyone was talking about Andrei Chemerkin. How much was he going to lift? Was he going to attempt a world record? Why was he competing in this meet? Was he even a university student? I joked to somebody that his college verification paperwork would probably be a cocktail napkin with the words "Andrei goes to school. Signed, Andrei" written on it in pencil. Although there was an entire world championship competition happening that weekend and, interestingly, a world record had been set in one of the lighter women's weight classes, the big Russian grizzly was the main event. After I flew into the airport and traveled to the hotel to check into my room, I turned around in the hotel lobby and saw him walking past me.

It's important to understand that this is one enormous piece of manflesh we're talking about. Andrei was walking near me and he paused for a few minutes to speak to somebody else, and I got a good look at him. His height wasn't overwhelming. I'm six feet tall and I was looking eye-to-eye with him. But the height wasn't what made the impression. This man's head looked like a cannonball. And believe me, that cannonball was sitting on top of a gargantuan pile of muscle. Andrei weighed around 175 kilos at the time (385 pounds, and we'll talk more about his bodyweight later). He was wearing sweatpants, a t-shirt, and a flannel jacket that looked like it could have functioned as a pup tent for a troop of Boy Scouts. I noticed that he had a pack of bananas jammed into his pocket as he walked away. I don't mean that he had two or three bananas, either. Think about when you go to the grocery store and you see the bananas in the produce section, with eight or nine of them attached in a bunch. Just pick up one of these bunches, without picking any of the bananas off, and ram it into your pocket. That's what I'm talking about.

A couple of days later, our competition was getting ready to start and the superheavyweights were in the warm-up room preparing to walk out on the platform for introductions. Our names were called and we were put in a line before the competition director walked us out to the platform. That's when I turned around and saw that it was happening the way I hoped it would... Andrei and I were right next to each other in the introduction line. Although I knew he didn't speak much English, I extended my hand to him and said, "Good luck today, brother." He smiled and shook my hand. Actually, I should say he swallowed my hand with his catcher's mitt of a paw. It was like shaking hands with the abominable snowman. When we walked out to the platform, the crowd went crazy. The announcer went down the line and introduced each athlete one-by-one, and the whole time I kept thinking to myself, "God, I hope somebody gets a picture of me standing next to him."

Side story: After the competition was over, I left Montreal to go home and I was convinced that nobody had taken a picture of us in the introduction line. It was a bummer because Andrei was a living legend and a picture of the two of us together would be a nice addition to my weightlifting scrapbook. I got home, a few weeks passed, and I got an envelope in the mail. Inside the envelope were two or three pictures from the competition, including a nice shot of Andrei and I standing side by side during the introductions. It was a total surprise to me when I got the pictures in the mail, and there was a note inside saying, "I was at this meet watching and I took these. I hope you like them!" The good Samaritan, who I didn't even know at the time, was a seventeen year-old lifter named Carissa Gordon. That's a true story.

Back to the meet...

I had a mediocre day on the platform and placed sixth in the superheavyweight class. Andrei won, obviously, with "light lifts" of 190 in the snatch and 230 in the clean and jerk. No world record attempts, but there was plenty to see and learn as I watched his every move during the competition. First of all, his "stretching routine" was quite a sight. After he put on his shoes, which he had to do by posting his foot against a chair and then leaning forward because his gut was too massive for him to reach his feet, he stood up. Then he hopped off the ground three or four times. And when I say "hopped," I mean he moved his girth up and down by bending and extending his knees. I'm not sure if his feet actually separated from the floor. Then he extended his arms out to his sides and shook his hands like he was trying to get water off them. Then he walked over to a bar loaded to seventy kilos and did his first set of snatches. So much for a thorough dynamic stretch routine prior to working out!

Aside from jokes about his mass and his stretching, it was easy to see why he was a great weightlifter as he progressed through his snatches. His technique was impeccable and every single lift looked exactly the same. Same positions, same speed, same apparent level of effort from seventy kilos all the way up to 170. His competition attempts were 180, 185, 190 and they looked exactly the same as the first set I had seen him do in the warm-up room. The strength of this man was mind-bending. Nothing changed about his attitude, his facial expression, or his state of calm. After the snatches were over, the C&J warm-ups started. This is where I got to see what so many people had talked about for the previous two years.

I'm referring to Chemerkin's clean and jerk technique. Beginning around 1997, Andrei had caused a lot of controversy in the weightlifting world because of a change in the way he performed the C&J. The basic explanation of it is that he no longer caught his cleans on his shoulders. He would go through the pulling movement of the clean and then, during the turnover phase, he would simply turn his wrists over and hold the bar about three inches off his shoulders. Imagine what it would look like if an athlete was holding a clean on their shoulders and then began to press the bar overhead. The position of the bar when it rose to the level of the Adam's apple, that's where Andrei held the bar in the cleans. He would stand up from the squat, go through the normal dip/drive of the jerk, and jerk the bar overhead for a completed lift. At no time during the lift had the bar touched his body, except for the hip drive during the pull. This was freaky to look at and it obviously contradicted a number of rules for proper weightlifting technique. Most people attributed the change in his technique to increased bodyweight. When Andrei won the 1996 Olympics, he weighed 165 kilos and his physique was relatively proportional. However, he began to add several kilos in the following years and, by the 1999 World Championship, he weighed 181 kilos (just under 400 pounds). Much of this additional mass had developed in his upper body. Because of the huge increase in the size of his shoulders and arms, he simply lost the flexibility to hold a clean on his shoulders.

Sounds like a problem, right? Most coaches would tell athletes in this position to lose some weight or do some stretching to fix the flexibility problem in their upper body. I mean, you have to be able to hold the bar on your shoulders to do a clean and jerk, correct? That's where the dilemma started with Chemerkin. This man, believe it or not, could clean and jerk around 250 kilos using this technique. It may sound unbelievable, but I stood next to the competition platform in Montreal that day when Andrei made his last C&J of 230 kilos, and I can positively verify that the bar never touched his shoulders. Not even in the jerk dip! He literally held the bar around the level of his chin through the entire lift. Right or wrong, it was a feat of strength from another universe. Moreover, he had been lifting like that since 1998 and he had continued to win world championships.

Despite the fact that his technique violated almost every rule of weightlifting (and physics), the man could still beat anybody on the planet. How could anybody tell him to fix anything?

TIME FOR SOME KIBITZING

In my humble opinion, Andrei fell victim to complacency during this process. He was the best lifter in the world and, for three years, nobody could touch him even if he was lifting with an atrocious technical error. Randall Strossen once approached him in the training hall of a world championship and asked him why he was clean and jerking this way. Chemerkin just smiled, pounded his shoulder with his fist and said, "Strong!" I believe the man saw himself as untouchable, regardless of any mistakes he was making. After his Atlanta victory, he did an interview with World Weightlifting magazine. In response to the question "What do you think of your future chances?" Andrei's response was, "I believe that at the next Olympic Games I will have an easier job than in Atlanta." He actually thought that his competition was going to get softer! However, we all know how this ride ended. A few months after Montreal, Andrei competed in the 2000 Sydney Olympics and got annihilated. Hossein Rezazedeh began his historic reign by winning the gold with a phenomenal 472.5 total. Ronny Weller, Chemerkin's former bridesmaid, won the silver with 467.5, and Armenian Ashot Danielyan won the bronze, leaving Chemerkin in fourth place. The untouchable champion had been shut out of the medals, completely. Eventually, Danielyan's drug test returned positive and he was forced to relinquish his bronze medal to Chemerkin. But regardless, it was a brutal thrashing for a man who many had thought was unbeatable.

So, what can we learn from this?

On the day of the Montreal competition, the sports page of the local newspaper featured an extensive interview with Chemerkin. The headline of the article was a quote from the champion that read, "The dream of everyone is to defeat me."

After the competition, a teammate of mine approached Andrei and gave him a USA weightlifting pin as a gesture of sportsmanship. Andrei took the pin, glanced at it, and then handed it to somebody else without even acknowledging my teammate.

The man was not modest or humble, or even gracious to his fellow competitors. These are qualities that are, for better or for worse, very common in great champions like Chemerkin. I've heard many stories about Vasily Alexeev that make Chemerkin sound like a contender for Miss Congeniality. Having a healthy dose of ego is an essential ingredient to being great at something. However, there is a caveat to it.

I believe Chemerkin became comfortable with the idea that nobody could beat him. Comfort is the enemy of progress. From my perspective, and this is just one man's opinion, that comfort level laid the foundation for some laziness. Now, can we call a man "lazy" if he is winning world championships? The answer to that question is YES because laziness begins as soon as the individual stops paying attention to all the little details. Some writers have referred to this concept as "believing your own headlines." Andrei's bodyweight increase, from 363 pounds when he won the gold medal in Atlanta to 400 pounds three years later, clearly did not work to his benefit. Basic understanding of physiology tells us that giant increases in body mass can potentially restrict flexibility, which is especially problematic in a sport that is as dependent on flexibility as weightlifting is. Andrei's upper-body flexibility went down the toilet and he continued to win world championships anyway, with snatches around 200 kilos and jerks around 260 kilos. But he did not make the training adjustments he needed to make to improve his total, and a hungry young Iranian lion was training Clubber Lang-style for the moment when he would have the chance to steal Chemerkin's claim to being the strongest weightlifter in the world. Andrei told a Montreal reporter that the dream of everyone was to defeat him. Those dreams became his worst nightmares before the summer of 2000 ended.

There are two final thoughts to this story. First of all, who am I to critique an Olympic gold medalist and three-time world champion? The man accomplished things that I never did, no doubt about it. This article, in a way, is the mother of all armchair quarterback articles. True, true... But despite these facts, I believe that there are lessons to be learned in everything and I sure as hell believe that the rise and fall of this particular weightlifter has some useful ones.

Second, competing against this colossus was one of the highlights of my career. Although I knew that I had no chance to beat him, it was still a privilege to share the stage with an athlete who had been to the absolute top of the mountain. Despite the fact that I think his career could have been different if he had taken more careful precautions with the flexibility problems he developed, there is still no doubt about the greatness of his career. Most athletes would sacrifice a limb to have one single moment when they can be identified as the best in the world. Andrei Chemerkin got to spend four years of his life in that moment. His performances were amazing. But, as Tom Hanks said, getting your butt kicked can make you better. Chemerkin kicked a lot of butts from 1997-1999. At the 1999 World Championship, he kicked Hossein Rezazedeh's butt. Then he went to the 2000 Olympics, the one he had predicted in the interview to be "easier than Atlanta." Apparently, Reza didn't get the memo. I guess weightlifting is like a box of chocolates. You never know what you're gonna get.

SO RUNS MY DREAM, BUT WHAT AM I?

Not long ago, an old friend of mine posted some information on the internet about using barbell exercises to strengthen and rehabilitate an athlete who had a severe problem with scoliosis. The story he posted was under the title "The healing power of the barbell."

That title caught my eye because it made me think about something from my own personal history in the iron game. When I first glanced at the words "the healing power of the barbell," I initially thought about the ways in which a person can be healed. Obviously, most of us think about healing in the context of injury recovery. We strain connective tissue, pull muscles, and tweak our bodies in a variety of different ways when we're fighting for bigger lifts and greater strength. Then our physiology has to heal and repair itself after these traumas. It's part of the game, nothing new to anybody.

However, that title took my brain in another direction. Aside from the physical aspect of it, I couldn't stop thinking about the idea of being healed in other ways. We go through times when we're frustrated or discouraged from lack of progress. We also experience defeats, either on the competition platform or in the bigger contest venue known as life. Some people walk through their lives carrying around scars and baggage from early experiences that were almost impossible to deal with in a positive way. And the thing we all have in common is that we all look for ways to heal ourselves after we've gone through hell. Some people pick destructive paths such as substance abuse or criminal activity because it seems like it will erase the pain, at least for a little while. Some people adopt pets. Some people learn to play a musical instrument. Some people submerge themselves in their professions or their relationships, thinking that constant focus on a certain area will eliminate any focus on the other areas that are difficult and depressing. Then, some people simply become bitter and vengeful because they want to build a brick wall around their soul and never give anybody else a chance to cause damage.

How does all of this connect to barbells? Seriously, how does all the Dr. Phil-type discussion lead us to a place where we can get some useful information out of this month's issue of *The Performance Menu*? Well... let me say a few words about that.

I love the 90s...

Aaahhh, 1998... I was twenty-six years old and at the top of my weightlifting game. My first Olympic weightlifting competition was in 1990. After spending a few years fumbling around in training and getting limited results, I decided to take this weightlifting thing all the way. I packed everything I owned into my 1981 Chevy Malibu station wagon, left my home in sunny Arizona, and drove up to rainy Washington so I could train for the legendary Calpian Weightlifting Club and be coached by John Thrush, the best weightlifting coach in America. The next five years of my life were brutal as I fought the weightlifting wars and attempted to work my way up the national rankings. Frustration? Plenty. Plateaus? Several. Best years of my athletic life? Absolutely, Jack.

Things started to pay off around 1997 because I moved up to superheavyweight from the 105 kilo class and my lifts shot up like a rocket. My breakout meet was the 1997 American Open in St. Joseph, Missouri where I snatched 150 and clean and jerked 180 for the first time, weighing under 120 kilos. For the next year and a half, I continued making progress and consistently won medals at all the top national meets in the United States. Times were fun. As H.I. McDonnough once said, they were the salad days.

However, lifting big weights and winning medals were only pieces of the entire puzzle. One of the best parts of being on the national weightlifting circuit was the friendships and bonds you formed with other lifters from around the country. This was always one of the elements of the lifting world that I loved the most. Even though one lifter lived in Florida and another lifter lived in Michigan and they only saw each other three or four times a year at national meets, it still felt like family. Everyone was around the same age, and the connection we all had through the sport we loved was an extremely tight link. I've always considered weightlifting a tribal sport, and being members of the tribe that competed at all the big meets made us brothers, sisters, cousins, and so on.

During these years, I ran with a crowd of lifters that liked to train hard and play hard. We were not choirboys. Maybe we would have been better weightlifters if we had played by the rules and spent all our post-competition time sitting in our hotel rooms and writing out our new weightlifting goals on Embassy Suites stationery, watching a Sandra Bullock movie and treating ourselves to a nice bowl of ice cream. I don't know for sure. What I do know for sure is that we liked going to bars, we liked drinking beer, we liked female companionship, we liked being young and strong, and we liked pushing the limits of safe, socially appropriate behavior. I'm surprised we didn't all grow up to become United States Congressmen.

One of my closest friends during this time was a lifter from Sacramento named Greg Johnson. Greg, like me, was a former football player-turned weightlifter and I think it's safe to say that he and I were sculpted from the same block of cheese. Along with Coach Bill Kutzer and a great pack of fellow weighlifters, Greg built the Team Sacramento Weightlifting Club from the ground up. Throughout the late 90s, Team Sac was consistently an impressive power at the national level. Their men's and women's teams were competitive, and the overall personality of their group was a lot like the Calpians. They had a coach who was a very good man and wanted nothing but the best for his lifters, who he treated like his own kids. They had a gang of athletes who trained hard, and they showed a noticeable enthusiasm and positive team attitude in all the things they did. We competed in all the same meets, we partied together, and we grew very close. Greg even had family in Washington State, so we would often see him a few times a year when he came to our gym to train while visiting. Although we lived in different areas, I considered Greg a brother in iron.

We all went through the salad days together. Down in the Sacramento area, Greg lifted, coached, and directed local meets that were fun and intense. Up in Washington, I did exactly the same thing with my club. The world was our oyster, and then things changed.

Losses...

As Jim Morrisson once said, "The future is uncertain and the end is always near."

On July 24th, 1999, I dislocated my knee during a 187.5 clean and jerk at a local meet in Auburn, Washington. It was less than a year before the 2000 Olympic Trials, which had been the ultimate goal of my career. Hell, it was the ultimate goal of my life. Weightlifting was practically my entire reason for breathing. I don't know if it was healthy or balanced to look at the world this way, but being a lifter was the most important thing in my existence. The Trials were around the corner, I was in the best shape of my life, and it was obvious from my training that much bigger lifts were about to fall. Now, I should mention that our 2000 Olympic Team consisted of only two men (who turned out to be Oscar Chaplin and Shane Hamman), and I knew I wasn't going to be in the mix for the top spots to go to Sydney. I was at 155/185 with the potential to maybe hit around 160/195, which clearly wasn't serious Olympic contention. But it didn't matter to me because from the time I first became a weightlifter, I knew that having the chance to compete in the Trials was a sacred honor that separated you from the pack in our sport, even if you didn't make the Olympic Team. I wanted it so bad, I couldn't stand it.

Then, when I had that 187.5 jerk over my head and I felt the bones in my knee separate, I knew it was all in jeopardy. It was a bad injury. After getting the MRI and speaking with a top surgeon, my options were clear. If I had surgery to repair the damage, I would be looking at almost a year of rehab. Or, I could skip the surgery and try to get back to my top lifts through strengthening the joint and physical therapy. The only choice I had to possibly make the Trials was option #2, clearly, so I skipped the surgery and started training again as soon as I could.

To make a long story short, I didn't get back to my top lifts after the injury and the 2000 Trials passed me by. My discouragement and disappointment were extreme, to say the least. In fact, I had practically decided to get out of Olympic weightlifting by 2001 because I couldn't stand the frustration. I spent the next three years squatting and deadlifting in the gym, only because I couldn't imagine my life without lifting weights. But there was no real focus, no real hope. I resigned myself to the idea that competing in the Olympic Trials was just something I was going to have to let go. This realization was like acid in my mouth, and I didn't handle it well at every given moment.

Then, the universe provided one of those moments when you snap to attention and look at everything just a little bit differently. I had been in the middle of a three-year pity party for myself when I woke up one day and found out that my old friend Greg Johnson, who I had continued to keep in touch with outside of weightlifting, had been killed in a car accident in early 2003.

It's an understatement to say Greg's death was an immensely painful blow to everyone who knew him. The news of his passing hit us like a hammer to the chest. He had a young son, he had recently been given a strength coaching position at Stanford University, and his hard work on the local weightlifting scene in California had nourished the sport in a valuable way. It was difficult for all of us to comprehend how such a bright light in the weightlifting world could be snuffed out so early. I think there are many people out there who still haven't come to terms with Greg's loss. It certainly made me ask some questions about life that I still don't know if I've found an answer for.

And a few months after it happened, his Team Sacramento family showed their typical classy character by announcing that there would be a Greg Johnson Memorial weightlifting meet in Sacramento in August of 2003. Just as Greg would have wanted it, the competition was going to be held on a beach, right next to the water, with loud music blasting and big weights flying. It was a chance for weightlifters to pay their respects to the memory of a good friend, and I made the decision that I was going to fly down and compete as soon as I heard about it. I had been out of competitive lifting for almost three years at the time. I had no plans to put together any kind of impressive total, and it didn't matter at all. What mattered was the having the chance to honor a fallen friend in the most appropriate way I could imagine, by lifting big weights on a platform with his name painted on it.

The 2003 Greg Johnson Memorial

When I arrived in Sacramento the day before the meet, it's fair to say that I was not exactly in the greatest phase of my lifting career. I had maintained some decent strength through the powerlifting movements I had been doing in the gym, but I wasn't ready to snatch or clean and jerk anything impressive. It had been almost a year since I had done a snatch in training. I had no idea what I could expect. And on top of all this, I had just gone through a very painful divorce. It wasn't the rock-bottom time period of my life, but it was a long way from the salad days.

Brett Kelly, Greg's close friend and Team Sac teammate, offered me a room in his house for the weekend. The day before the meet, all the volunteers got together to haul the weights, platform lumber, and meet supplies to the beach and set up for the next day. I wanted to be in on all of it, regardless of how tired it made me for the meet the next day. We all worked until sundown to prepare the competition area, and then we went out to eat burgers, drink beers, and tell Greg stories. When the meet began the next day, there was something in the air. In twenty years of weightlifting, I don't think I've ever seen a competition where there was as much happiness, enthusiasm, mutual support, and weightlifting ca-maraderie as there was at this meet. To put it simply, everything was perfect. The sun was shining, people were smiling and lifting with everything they had, the music was blasting, and lots of fans had showed up to watch the action. In other words, it was exactly the way Greg would have wanted it.

And the crazy part of the whole experience is that I had an incredible day of lifting. I went three-for-three in the snatch, nailing an easy 142.5 on my last at-tempt. In the clean and jerk, I made 155, 165, and cleaned 170 for a narrow miss in the jerk. These weights were still well below my personal bests, but they were much better than I had expected. However, more important than the weights I lifted was the way I felt on the platform. I felt the energy of this meet in my bone marrow. I felt the spiritual presence of a lost friend who gave everything he had to make people better weightlifters, and all the smiles and laughs we had shared as we sat on barstools and toasted the prime years of our youth. I felt the disap-pointment and pain from the last three years of my life melting off me like frost every time I chalked my hands and stepped on the platform. I howled at the sky like an animal after successful lifts. People were screaming, "Do it for Greg!!" as I reached down to grip the bar and I knew, for some reason, that all of my pathetic little problems were no bigger than the molecules of dust that rose from the plat-form when the bumper plates came crashing down. This moment... this perfect moment was a healing experience for me. The loss of my weightlifting dream and the loss of my marriage evaporated into the air of that beach as I held that barbell over my head. After my last lift, with the applause and appreciation of the weightlifting family still ringing out, I took off my weightlifting shoes, ran off the platform, and dove into the cool water. The waves rippled as I rose to the surface and floated on my back for a few minutes, looking at the blue sky and listening to the meet announcer laughing into the microphone and thanking the crowd for coming out to watch the meet. I can tell you right now, seven years later, that it was one of the happiest moments of my life.

I got out of the water, dried off, and Brett started handing out the awards to the athletes. The biggest award of the day was an enormous trophy that had "The Greg Johnson Memorial Award" engraved on the plate. Team Sacramento

MATT FOREMAN

had designed the award to be given to the athlete who, as they phrased it, demonstrated spirit and intensity on the platform that would honor Greg Johnson's memory. They gave me this trophy, and it stands on a cabinet in the den of my house. I'm looking at it as I type these very words.

The aftermath...

When I came home from this competition, I had the fire back in my guts. I was encouraged by the lifts I had been able to make at the meet and it occurred to me that I wanted to give my weightlifting career another shot. Four months later, I won the silver medal at the American Open. Four months after that, I placed fourth at the Senior National Championships and qualified to compete in the 2004 US Olympic Trials at the age of 32.

In a twist of poetic justice, I traveled back to good old St. Joseph, Missouri for the Trials. My knee was hurting, training hadn't gone perfect, I had no realistic shot of actually making the Olympic Team, and I didn't give a damn about any of these things. With the help of a departed friend, I had dug myself out of a black pit of self-doubt, and I stood on the Olympic Trials competition platform with my final clean and jerk completed over my head. Somebody in St. Joseph must have known something about my comeback situation because after my lifting session was over and the fans had all left the auditorium, the name "Foreman" stayed illuminated on the scoreboard. I found a chair, sat down next to the platform, and stared at that scoreboard until the custodial crew told me that they were shutting off the lights and locking the building up. Then I went back to the meet hotel, cleaned up, and went to meet some old friends for beers.

I've spent a lot of time since the 2004 Trials thinking about how this whole story unfolded. Greg Johnson's death was a tragedy that nothing can cure. It made my knee injury and personal problems look like a game of tiddlywinks. Many of you who are reading this article have felt your share of dark moments just like these. Certainly, some of you have even walked through hellfire that was much hotter than anything I've spoken of. You might even be feeling the flames of those fires right now. And I don't have any magic words for you that are going to fix anything. Nobody does. All I can offer is the idea that there is a healing out there somewhere, and it probably lies in the thing you love most. After all the years of frustration, my healing came from doing the most obvious thing I could think of... going back to weightlifting. Weightlifting was what I loved most, and my salvation had been right in front of my face the whole time. Maybe we're all part of a bigger plan, and that plan is going to drag us over some rough territory at times. Maybe there is no plan, and everything that happens to us in life is just random activity.

Either way, there are a few things I know for sure. Life is a beautiful thing, the world is a fine place, and the best thing we can all do is try to find love and happiness while we've still got the chance. The title of this article is a line from a poem by Alfred, Lord Tennyson. He wrote it after his best friend died in 1833. The last line I'll give you is from Bob Marley:

"Everything's gonna be all right."

SECTION THREE: GENERAL ATHLETIC EXPERIENCE

Many of you are coaches. You should consider yourself lucky if you can hold this title, because coaching is one of the best jobs in the world. It's also one of the toughest, especially if you hang in it for years and decide to make a career out of it.

I've coached several different sports and a wide range of age groups. Coaching is a people profession, and the people are what I remember most from my years of doing this. Sure, it's nice to have your teams win championships and your athletes win medals. We're all competitive people, and we want to reach the top of our fields. But when I think about what I've loved most about sports, it's the daily process of working together, training hard, and sharing a big part of my life with other special people. I hate to resort to quotes that have been used a million times, but there is one that I think applies to this section pretty well:

"The goal is not the end of the road. The goal is the road."

THE ANSWERS ARE
BETWEEN YOUR EARS

What can I learn from this?

That's the question I found myself asking over and over when I read William Faulkner's novel *The Sound and the Fury*. I teach American Literature for a living, I love books, Faulkner is generally considered one of the greatest American writers ever and this novel is his landmark accomplishment, so it seemed like a perfect choice when I picked it off the shelf of a used bookstore in Tacoma, Washington many years ago. The problem is that it's not an easy read. *The Sound and the Fury* is written using "stream of consciousness" technique, which is where the writer tells a story through the internal thought process of a character. It's tricky to keep up with stories that are told in this manner, and Faulkner's novel makes it even tougher because the whole first section of the novel is written stream-of-consciousness through the eyes of a mentally handicapped man named Benjy Compson.

We're going to try something a little different in this month's article. We're going to examine your personal experience as strength athletes. The writing is going to be mostly about you, there are going to be a lot of rapid fire questions that you're going to answer in your mind as you read, and all of this is going to be pointed towards learning some kind of lesson that's going to make you a better coach or athlete. This is going to be borderline stream-of-consciousness writing, and your job is simply to follow along. Now, I'm going to make it a little easier on you than William Faulkner made it on me. I'm going to stop at the end of the article and ask the question, "What's the point?" And because I want you to feel like you're getting your money's worth out of your *Performance Menu* subscription, I'll go ahead and tell you what the point is when we get there. Knowing that you're all brainy people, you'll probably have the underlying message of the article figured out long before I spoon feed it to you. Maybe this will be a literary accomplishment that rivals Faulkner, who knows? Maybe one of you will want to nominate me for the Nobel Prize in literature. Or maybe you'll finish this article and think I'm as mentally handicapped as Benjy Compson. You probably wouldn't be the first to arrive at that conclusion.

Let's talk about you.

Where are you going, where have you been?

First of all, think about what you are. Are you an Olympic weightlifter? Are you a powerlifter? Are you a general strength trainer? Are you a Crossfitter? Are you a coach, in addition to one of these other things? Try to assign yourself a certain title. If you participate in a lot of different strength disciplines or roles, which one is most important to you? Just think... if you had to stand up and introduce yourself like addicts do at recovery meetings, where they say "My name is _____, and I'm an alcoholic," what would your classification be? Some of you might just want to call yourselves LIFTERS. That's fine.

How long have you been doing what you're doing as a strength athlete? I'm talking about sustained, focused practice on this particular area that you identified. Who taught you how to do it? Were you self-taught? What would you consider your top accomplishment so far? Think about the high points of what you've done. What your top lifts are, what competitions you've participated in, things like that. If you had to sit down with a pen and paper and write down your number one most significant achievement in your area, what would it be? Take a minute if you need to, and figure out what it is. Don't go on reading until you have something specific isolated in your mind. It might be a one-rep max in one of the Olympic lifts, it might be a championship you've won, it might be a team or athlete you've coached or a gym you've built from the ground up.

When you know what your top achievement is, file it away in your brain and remember it. Once you've done that, I want you to shift gears slightly and think about the people you train with or compete against on a regular basis. These might be the people in your gym. They might be lifters or athletes from around the state, nation, or world. Maybe you have a particular rival, somebody you could point out as being your top competitor. Maybe you hate this person. Maybe you love them. Maybe you think about them when you put your hands on a bar and prepare for a big set, whispering their name as motivation to grind out your reps. Maybe this person doesn't even know who you are, and it's your goal to make sure they learn your name and can't forget it somewhere down the road. Or perhaps this doesn't apply to you very well because you don't really feel like you're in competition with anybody, which is fine too. In that case, just think about other people who train in the same area as you.

Now, go back to your top accomplishment from a few moments ago. Remember it? Okay, now put it together with the people you just named as your competitors, training partners, peers, or whatever. And ask yourself this big question... *How do you stack up against others?* Are you the best in your area? Maybe you're the best in your gym, but not in your state. Maybe you're one of the top two or three in the country, with only a couple of names who are better than you. Maybe you're a world champion. Be totally honest when you rank yourself. Don't lie and don't make excuses. If you're the weakest lifter in your gym, then just come right out and say it. Make sure you put yourself on a level playing field, by the way. If you're a 140-pound woman and you train in a gym full of 220-pound guys, don't classify them as your peers. Think about the people who are directly comparable to you. If you're a coach, how does your athlete production compare to the other coaches you know? Make sure you have a solid idea about where you stand in relation to others before you move on to the next paragraph.

Got it figured out? Okay, so how do you feel about where you are? Take a second and tell yourself the truth. Are you happy with what you've done at this point? Do you feel a sense of pride and self-confidence in your status? Do you feel like you've accomplished some of your biggest goals, or are you on the other end of the spectrum? Do you feel embarrassed, like everybody is ahead of you and you're ashamed of it? Do you consider your accomplishments unimpressive or below average compared to your peers? Are you angry at other people because of your own predicament?

More importantly, how much of your potential do you think you've reached? Do you think you've used absolutely every ounce of gas you have in your tank? Have you squeezed every drop out of your lemon? If the answer to this question is no, then what has stopped you? Why haven't you reached the heights you know you could get to? For some of you, it might just be an issue of time. You might be saying to yourself that you know you're capable of a 300-pound clean and jerk and the only reason you haven't reached it yet is because you've only been training for six months and you're still working your way up the ladder. That's acceptable. Hopefully, most of you fit that description. Hopefully, there's not a darker reason why you're not getting maximum results from yourself, like laziness or fear.

This next part might sting just a little bit. I want you to think about somebody who does the same thing you do (Olympic lifter, Crossfitter, etc.), but I want you to specifically think about somebody who is better than you despite the fact that they've only been training for a short period of time. Let's go back and look at some of our previous questions for an example. If you said earlier that you've been training as a lifter for three years and your top achievement is a 275-pound clean, I want you to think of somebody you know who has only been training for nine months and has already cleaned 315 at the same bodyweight as you (or lighter). This person has less experience than you, and they've already been able to accomplish more than you have. Don't apply any smoke-and-mirrors excuses to this section. You need to pinpoint somebody who has passed you by, despite the fact that they haven't put in as much time and work as you.

Intermission/personal example I started Olympic lifting in 1990. At the 1998 Senior National Championship, I snatched 330 pounds and clean and jerked 402 pounds in the superheavyweight class. At the time, this was my best competition ever, my highest accomplishment. At this contest, Shane Hamman snatched 385 pounds and clean and jerked 462 in the same weight class as me. I believe he had only been training as an Olympic lifter for around two years at that point. I had been working much longer than he had, and his accomplishments surpassed mine by a country mile. This is the type of situation I want you to personalize.

End of intermission.

It's bothersome to think about this, no doubt about it. The thing that makes this bothersome is when you simply have to admit that somebody else is more talented than you. Despite the fact that you've invested a greater time commitment and workload, this other person is going to move ahead of you and enjoy greater rewards than you've been able to taste. The thing that makes you angry is that this doesn't seem fair. The normal perceptions of justice indicate that the people who work the hardest and the longest should be the people who receive the greatest blessings. But the world of strength athletics, like most other areas of our universe, is not based on fairness. If you want justice, look in the dictionary between jerky and juxtapose.

One of the things that can make this whole thing even more irritating is if the person who has moved ahead of you has a detestable personality. When you get beaten by a newbie and that newbie happens to be a mouthy punk, it'll feel like needles under your toenails. What if your strength training is one of the biggest parts of your life? What if it's THE biggest part of your life? And despite how much you love it and how much you've sacrificed for it, some scumbag with a big mouth is tasting the good life while you get relegated to the back of the bus.

Maybe you don't know what I'm talking about. Maybe you've never dealt with this and your attitude about your training life is completely different from how I'm describing things. Maybe none of this frustration applies to you at all. If that's the case, good for you. You live in a place called Happyland. And I want you to fully enjoy every aspect of Happyland, truly. But go ahead and read the rest of this article anyway, just in case Happyland is ever invaded by the aforementioned mouthy punks and you have nowhere to run.

Tomorrow and tomorrow and tomorrow...

Where do we go from here? What can we learn from any of this? Now that you've got a mental image of a competitor who is more talented than you and you're nice and agitated, what's the next angle to look at? Why have we spent this time examining ourselves, and how can any of this make us better lifters or coaches? For crying out loud, WHAT'S THE POINT?

Stay with me for a few more minutes. Answer some more questions, and we'll get to the bottom line soon. First of all, why did you get into the strength game to begin with? What did you want to accomplish? What results were you looking for? Try to come up with a legitimate answer to this. Once you have the answer, ask yourself another question. Did you think those results were going to come to you quickly? Did you think the path you chose was going to be easy? How long did you plan to commit to these goals of yours? Did anybody explain to you, right from the very beginning, that the pursuit of those goals might turn into a lifelong journey? Are you even interested in a lifelong journey? How much do you love what you do?

Now, let's build up to the climax moment of our little self-exploration. Ask yourself one question, just one tiny little question that should lead to an enormous answer: *What can you start doing that will make your journey more successful?* Instead of focusing on other athletes and how much weight they're lifting, turn the focus back towards yourself and examine what you can do to make yourself better. Forget about what other people have. What do YOU have, inside yourself, and what can you do to make forward progress? Obviously, the most immediate answers to this question involve training-related issues. Better training programs, better injury rehab/prehab measures, better dietary practices, better hydration, better sleep scheduling, better learning about the techniques of your sport. Look at all of these topics and figure out how much attention you're giving to each of them. As soon as you finish this article, you should sit down with a pen and paper. Make a list of the ten most important aspects of your training life. Then, next to each one of those aspects, give yourself a personal score on a scale of one through ten. A score of ten means that you're really putting complete concentration and effort into that area, and a score of one means that you basically don't take it seriously at all. Give yourself the most honest answers you're capable of, and then ask yourself this question again: *What can you start doing that will make your journey more successful?*

And I guess I want to finish this article by going one step further, one more step beyond the focus on training issues like stretching, nutrition, and programming. I want you to think about your personality. Think about your life. I want you to ask the big question for a third time, what can you start doing that will make your journey more successful? But now, I want you to apply that question to areas like your self-concept, your attitude, how you interact with others, how much enthusiasm you demonstrate in your life, how many positive things you do or say for somebody else on a daily basis, how often you tell people that you appreciate them. Do you hold the door open for other people when you're walking into a gas station? Do the most important people in your life know how much they mean to you? Do your training partners feel more energetic and excited when you're in the gym? If you have people in your life that you love, do you tell them that? If you're a coach, do your athletes respect you and want to fight their hardest for you? When you think about your future, do you focus on obstacles and negative possibilities? Or do you imagine the great moments of triumph that could happen if you take some risks and strengthen your work ethic?

William Faulkner, like a lot of great writers, was a big drinker. He would stay sober while he was writing, and then go on powerful benders when he was finished. The characters in *The Sound and the Fury* were members of a formerly successful Southern family who struggle to cope with their lives as they watch their family's greatness crumble over the years. Despite the brilliance of the writer and the inspiration of what he produced, there is a dark streak to his body of work. We're going to turn that dark streak in the opposite direction when we finish this reading. We're going to walk away from this article and start looking for ways to train better, live better, and feel better. We're going to think of things that will make us happy, because happiness makes your lifts go up. How many things did you do yesterday that made your life better? Honestly, make a mental list right now. When you're done, think of six things you can do with the rest of this day that will make you a better athlete and a better person.

Once you've figured out what those things are, go out and do them.

OUR LITTLE FURRY FRIENDS

Most of the people I know love dogs and hate cats.

Sure, there are exceptions to everything. I know there are a few odd ducks out there who aren't crazy about dogs, and we certainly understand that the world has its share of cat people. But if I took a poll of everybody I meet on a daily basis, I would venture a guess that the majority of them would favor the puppies over the felines. Personally, I love them both, and one of the things that never stops interesting me is watching the personality differences between the two. Let me give you an example of what I'm talking about. Imagine a moment when you bring one of these animals into a new house that it's unfamiliar with. First, think about what the dog will do. As soon as that pooch gets through the front door, he will start running around the house to check everything out. He wants to jump on every couch, sniff every plant, investigate every room, and just generally have a wild and crazy exploring session with his tail wagging hard enough to knock over every picture frame in the place. He's excited, and he has no fear of anything.

Then, I want you to think about what happens when you do the exact same thing with a cat. For those of you who haven't brought a cat into a new house, let me tell you how it goes. Most of the time, the kitty is going to get pretty cautious as soon as he realizes that he's in a new environment. He will walk low to the ground, move slowly, and most likely look for a bed or something that he can crawl under and hide as quickly as possible. It will probably take at least a few days for the cat to start getting comfortable with exploring the house and being sociable with new people. Cats are just like that, plain and simple.

The thing that I really find fascinating is how these basic differences in behavior can also be applied to athletes. When you work with people in a setting of athletic training and competition, you can definitely see which ones are "dogs" and which ones are "cats." Some people have character traits that are more similar to Fido, while others are the walking talking versions of Garfield. As a coach, these differences become more and more clear as time goes on. The behaviors you see in this regard will determine how the athlete approaches daily workouts, competition, and every other aspect of what you do in the gym. If you want to be a successful coach, you need to know how to handle each one effectively. Coaching is not a one-size-fits-all profession. Athletes have to be talked to and handled differently if they're all going to reach their maximum potential. Failure to comply with this notion can leave you with an empty gym, so let's take this month's article and see if we can come up with some useful information about how to manage the pet population of your training world.

Bow wow wow, yippee yo yippee yay

The first athlete personality we're going to examine is the dogs. When we talk about athletes who fit the dog temperament, we're talking about the ones who are high on aggression and low on fear. These are the lifters who will go 100% hell-bent-for-leather in every single workout if you let them. They'll attack their workouts the same way that dog will attack his new house investigation. Typically, the dog athletes have a fierce enthusiasm for training and are willing to do anything you tell them to do... and more. If you want them to attempt a personal record six or seven times in a workout, they'll do it. In fact, they'll probably keep attempting it until you tell them to stop, and even then they'll argue with you because they just KNOW they can hit that snatch on the fourteenth try. You often have to run them out of the gym at the end of the day because they'll keep going until you shoo them away.

Dog athletes aren't scared of much. The idea of failing in an attempt or possibly even getting injured just doesn't seem to enter into their minds. To them, the whole training experience is just like a golden retriever going to a dog park for the day with a master who has tons of tennis balls and all the time in the world. And like the dog with the tennis ball, these athletes like to challenge you. If you've ever played fetch with a dog, you've probably noticed how the dog brings the tennis ball back to you after you throw it, but he also makes you fight to take the ball out of his mouth before you can throw it again. He likes to battle you a little bit. You have to grip the ball and really pull to get it out of his teeth, and he's not giving it up easily. He's not doing this because he wants to keep the ball and end the fetch game. Believe me, he wants you to take the ball away from him because he wants you to throw it again. He just likes the playfulness of grappling with you. Dog athletes are the same way. They're going to scuffle with you in the gym sometimes.

For example, there might be a situation where the athlete wants to work up and try a max attempt in the back squat because he/she is feeling good that day, but you (the coach) don't want him/her to do any max squat attempts because you've planned some near-maximum snatch attempts for the following day and you don't want their legs to get too fatigued. This might bring about a little back-and-forth exchange between you and the athlete about who is going to make the final decision. At this point, you have to make the decision on how stern you want to be with your treatment of the athlete. If you blow a gasket and verbally explode on them, it might cause your entire relationship to take a turn for the worse. The athlete might walk away from the tongue-lashing like a dog would walk away from being kicked, and you don't want that. When it's all said and done, you still want both the dog and the athlete to feel empowered and enthusiastic. Of course, there is always a chance that you might be working with a turbocharged headstrong athlete who simply won't obey your instructions *unless* you verbally explode on them. These athletes are exhausting to work with because they make you ride them like a pack mule day after day. You have to practically beat them with a hammer to get them to obey, and you have to make your own call about whether it's worth it to you to keep butting heads with them over and over. If the constant combat is wearing you down, tell them to get out of the gym for a while and decide whether they want to train on your terms or not.

However, there are plenty of obvious positives about dog athletes. If you can get them under control, they have a much better chance of becoming successful because of their natural intensity and willingness to work hard. Laziness won't be much of an issue here. And as with dogs, these athletes will often develop a powerful loyalty to you as they grow and develop. Through smart discipline and intelligent treatment, you will wind up with a lifter who is not only a well-trained weightlifting machine, but also willing to chew somebody's leg off if they give you any trouble. It's a good feeling when you reach this stage.

Hello Kitty

In my opinion, most of the athletes you work with in weightlifting will be dog athletes. This is simply because a person has to have some dog in them to even give weightlifting a try in the first place. This sport requires a lot of courage, even if the lifter isn't planning to compete. Most people in the world jump out of the way when they see a heavy iron weight falling towards the ground. Weightlifters jump under it and try to catch it. That tells you something about what kind of people we are.

Still, regardless of the basic principles of weightlifting and what kind of personality they lend themselves to, there are going to be plenty of potential trainees coming into your gym who have a little more of the cat qualities we hinted at earlier. First and foremost, cat athletes will be much more cautious than dog athletes. I hesitate to use the words "fearful" or "scared" because these terms both carry a negative connotation, and it's important for a coach to always see athletes in a positive way. So cat athletes will be very hesitant about stepping out of their comfort zones. They will often have a particular amount of weight that they are comfortable attempting in workouts, something they know they can make consistently with very little chance of failure. And it won't be easy to get them to load a few more kilos on the bar and take a shot at it. You (the coach) will have to push them to attempt new personal records. They won't instinctively go for it on their own. Also, they will often take a long time to warm up to you or demonstrate any loyalty, much like cats.

These athletes instinctively avoid situations that could result in pain, embarrassment, or failure. And it is worth mentioning that many coaches simply won't bother working with athletes who demonstrate cat qualities in the early stages. Coaches will dismiss these athletes as cowards and simply conclude that they just don't have the mental disposition to be weightlifters. This is where it would be wise to step back and examine some more productive ways to work with the cat athletes. Weightlifting is a small sport, and it's not easy to find people who are willing to seriously pursue it. If you're lucky enough to train somebody who has legitimate enthusiasm and desire to snatch, clean, and jerk, then it is worth your time to think of some interpersonal techniques that will keep this person around and give them a chance to be successful. Even if they are timid and hesitant about taking risks, there are still ways to work with them. Mainly, the coach has to find a way to push the athlete while still providing a sense of safety. Often, the cat athletes will be reluctant to attempt personal records simply because they feel like they will disappoint the coach if they fail. As a coach, you have to make it clear to the athlete that you are supportive of them even if they don't always succeed. Basic expressions like "we'll get it next time" or "I'm proud of your effort" can go a long way. Cats don't come out from under the bed when they get screamed at. They come out from under the bed when they're confident in their surroundings.

Now, is it also possible for an athlete to be such a basket case personality that they're basically impossible to work with? Absolutely, and I've seen a few of these. There might come a time when you (the coach) have to tell an athlete to hit the bricks in order to avoid losing your other athletes because they won't train in the same gym as the wacko. My personal experience is that these types are few and far between, but you never know. Some cats have lived in a dysfunctional home for so long that they're beyond socialization. They just need their own cage, plain and simple.

It's also worth mentioning that cats can be very dangerous when they feel trapped or defensive. Try dealing with a cat sometime when its ears are pointed backwards, its back is arched, and you can hear it making a growling noise. If you try to pick that cat up and scold it at that moment, be prepared to walk away with some scratches on your face.

Species Identification

Where do you fit in this discussion? Look at yourself from the outside and think about which animal you most closely relate to. How about your coaches? Would they say you're a dog or a cat?

Looking back at myself as a young weightlifter, I think I was a pretty direct example of a dog athlete. I grew up in a small town where the high school weight room was the only place to train. It was a free standing building behind the football stadium, and it was always locked during non-school hours. I didn't have time in my schedule to take a weight training class, so I used to go there at five o'clock in the morning and pick the lock on the back door so I could get inside and train by myself with no heat, almost no lighting, and no coaching. Then I had to get out of there before the teachers showed up and busted me for breaking in.

I wanted to be a lifter, and nothing was going to stop me from doing it. When I finally hit the big time and moved to a gym where I had a coach, I was not easy to handle. I wanted to go as heavy as I could every single day, and I had no problems with trying a personal record twelve times in a row. I also had a defiant attitude and a short fuse, which didn't make me the world's most endearing young trainee. In retrospect, I have to thank God that I had a coach who didn't get fed up and kick me out of the gym. He certainly had reason to. But as I've mentioned in this article, he found a way to condition me to his way of doing things. To use some dog terminology, he had to swat me in the nose with a rolled up newspaper and rub my snout in my own mess a few times. And he did it in a way that let me know he wanted me to be successful and he didn't hate me. As time passed, I learned. I learned who the boss was, and I learned that following his instructions was going to put me in a better position to be a champion. After a few years, my loyalty to him was so strong that I would have chewed broken glass if he told me to.

You have to learn the same methods, and then you have to develop your own style of conditioning your athletes to follow your methods. It takes time, believe me. Coaching is a skill that takes a long time to develop, just like athletic prowess. But you'll be okay if you remember that people have differences, and they require different treatment. If you don't believe me, put your cat on a leash and try to take it for a walk around the block the same way you would with a dog. See how that works for you.

SUCKS TO YOUR ASS-MAR

The next time you think about getting depressed because you've got some kind of physical ailment or you're in a position where you're being treated unfairly, think about this. Tommy Kono is probably one of the greatest weightlifters ever, an American who won two Olympic gold medals in 1952 and 1956. Tommy had a difficult time participating in sports when he was a young child because he had asthma. During World War II, Tommy's family was relocated to a Japanese internment camp in Tule Lake, California. During this time, the dry climate cured Tommy's asthma and he was able to begin learning weightlifting. He went on to become the best in the world. If you've got something wrong with you or you're getting screwed over, remember that those situations might be the foundation of some mental strength that's going to take you far in life.

THE FOUR PHASES
OF WEIGHTLIFTING

Have you ever stopped and thought about how so many things in life happen in different stages? Almost anything you can think of in your life probably followed some kind of progression; it happened in a phase one, phase two, phase three kind of order. Let's look at a really easy example to make this more understandable. Many of you are in long-term relationships, right? Some of you are married, and others have had a boyfriend or girlfriend for an extended period of time. I know this has to be true because people who read Performance Menu are generally smarter and more attractive than non-readers, so we usually don't stay single for very long.

Your relationship with your significant other has developed in stages. Think back about the time period when you originally met this person and started going out on your first dates. Think about how you acted, how you talked, how you dressed, etc. Most likely, you were on your best behavior and trying to look extra hot because you wanted something to happen with this person. You cleverly concealed any personal glitches of yours that other people might find gross because you were on a mission to look as tantalizing as possible. That was stage one. Then, there was a time when you two decided that you were an actual couple, and the newness of the relationship started to wear off. You got used to each other, and you got to discover some wonderfully special personal habits your partner has. Some of these were charming and funny, while many others were probably disgusting and irritating. That was stage two, and many couples never make it through this one. Lots of casualties in this area.

If you decided that this person's lifestyle was something you could live with, then you might have even progressed to stage three. This is where you're serious, and you start talking and planning serious future type of stuff. You think about getting married and buying houses. Once you're in this stage, it's intense business. You're considering spending the rest of your life with this person, and that's pretty heavy stuff to think about. Nervousness and second thoughts are common here. Some couples stick it out, and some don't.

So... that brings us to weightlifting and strength training. You might not even know it, but your experience as a weightlifter has also happened in stages. This also true for all the people you coach, if you're a coach. What I want to do this month is take a look at the stages of a lifter's career, and all the different variables that accompany these stages. If you coach lifters, you need to have an understanding of what's going through their minds when they come into your gym. Because if you're oblivious to the thoughts and concerns of your athletes, there's a strong chance that misunderstandings and conflicts will pop up. These can make gym life pretty sticky, and they could even lead to a break-up. Just like your life with your special little love interest, it's pretty damn important to be able to see things not just from your own perspective, but from theirs, too. Mutual understanding will almost always make things easier, whether you're talking about snatching a personal record or shopping for an engagement ring. So, let's take a look at the stages that you, your athletes, and every other person who calls themselves a weightlifter will go through during your relationship with the barbell.

Stage One: Clueless Rookie

Even though the term "clueless rookie" carries a negative tone, this first stage of your weightlifting life is one of the most exciting times you'll ever get to feel. This is when you are brand spanking new to the iron world. You may or may not have had some athletic experience at this point and you might have even done some form of weight training, but the focused discipline of serious weightlifting training is a whole new ball game. You don't really know anything about weightlifting at this point, but you do know for sure that you're interested in it. You're full of energy and curiosity. This is when you're first learning the snatch, clean and jerk, or maybe the squat or deadlift if you're a powerlifter instead of an Olympic lifter. Every day that you come to the gym is a new experiment of teaching your body to do something that it has never done. Frustration is guaranteed at this point, no questions asked. The complexity of the Olympic lifts are challenging for even the most talented natural athletes. You probably get to wipe out in some creative way in this stage, either through nailing your chin with the bar in the jerk, falling on your butt when jumping under a snatch, or some other wacky accident. Veterans, do you remember those days? You got embarrassed because there were probably other people in the gym who were experienced lifters and you felt like genetic sludge when you biffed it in front of them. Hey, this is like the awkward stage children have to go through. You're like the little boy who came to school and found out the hard way that the cool kids don't pull their pants all the way down around their ankles when they pee at the urinal.

But the great thing about this phase is that you also get to have those moments when everything clicks. You hit your first snatch correctly, and you FEEL the proper movement for the first time in your life. If I could offer a word of advice to coaches at this point...make sure you celebrate and compliment your newbies when they have little technique breakthroughs. Even though they might still have five or six technical glitches that need to get fixed and they're a long way from perfect, you have to remember that it's very important for new lifters to feel like they're making some kind of progress. Even if it's the smallest of baby steps, make your people feel like they're moving forward. That's what will keep them coming back for more. I've seen aspiring new lifters quit the sport because their coaches were such perfectionists that they basically wouldn't give ANY positive feedback in this phase.

If you're the lifter, please try to remember that this phase will be rough. You're going to have little aches and pains in places that you never have before. You're going to have moments when you feel like you've mastered the technique of a lift and then, three days later, you lose that mastery and feel like you forgot how to lift correctly. The aggravation is going to be a part of this stage, but that aggravation is a good thing. If you get angry when you do something wrong, that means it's important to you. You have a hungry spirit, and you get pissed when you fail because you really, really want to be good at this. That's the right attitude, believe me. The people who don't care if they make progress are the ones who will never amount to jack squat because their performance doesn't mean anything to them. Just hang in there, baby.

Stage Two: Turbo Teenager

Whoa daddy! At this point, you've passed the rookie phase and now you're moving up in the world. Stage two is when you're no longer a newbie and you've actually started to perfect the lifts and make progress. In fact, you've probably made enormous progress in a short period of time. The Olympic lifts are very difficult to learn, but the athlete will make remarkable gains during the time when the technique has clicked and strength improvements have begun.

This is when you've been lifting for maybe a year, or possibly even two or three years. Now, you actually do know some stuff about weightlifting. You understand the technique of the lifts and the training process. You've lifted some solid weights, too. You can probably even beat many of the other lifters around you. This is when many of you have begun competing, and you now have some meets under your belt. You might have even competed at the national level. This is a great time because you're good at weightlifting and you know it. Most likely, you've even started to teach others. Full-time coaching probably hasn't become your thing yet because you're climbing the ladder as an athlete. But you've helped some people with their technique in the gym, or even taught some beginners who are in stage one, just like you were not too long ago. The stage one people look at you as an expert because you can lift a lot more than they can, which boosts your pride and self-image. Basically, things are awesome at this point.

However, there is one thing about this stage that can be funky. What am I talking about? I'm talking about the fact that you probably think you know every freaking thing there is to know about weightlifting at this point. Trust me, stage two is when you start to get pretty big for your britches. Because you're now a qualified weightlifter, you start to think that your expertise is a lot bigger than most of the people out there. This is when you get on the internet and argue with people about weightlifting because you're right and they're wrong, dammit. That's why this stage is called the "turbo teenager" stage. You're like a seventeen year-old kid who thinks they know everything about life. You don't want to listen to your parents because you think they're old, out of touch with reality, and they don't have a clue about what your life is like. You've got enough hormones pumping through your body to fuel an oil tanker, and you won't back down from a fight.

At this point, you think the best weightlifters are the biggest experts on weightlifting. That's how you see it. And let me say a word to the coaches at this point. This stage two will be a blessing and a curse, just like being a parent and raising teenagers. The blessing of this stage is that your athletes will do a lot of incredible things that make you very proud. They're developing quickly, and it's a lot of fun to guide them while they blast away new personal records and rise up into the higher ranks of the sport. However, the curse is that they'll be hard to handle, just like the teenagers. They're going to say stupid things that piss you off. They're going to disobey you and violate the rules you've asked them to live by. They're going to require some tough love if you want them to remember that you're the authority figure and you're still in charge of this operation. Don't be afraid to lay down the law here. You're going to have to do it anyway, and most athletes respond well when they know they're following an alpha.

Stage Three: Holy crap, you mean I'm human?

Now, things are tough. Stage three occurs when you've had some years of experience under your belt. You've risen to a high level and you have some legitimate accomplishments on your record. You can look back on what you've done so far and feel a sense of reward, but now there's a problem.

Stage three is when something has happened to knock you down. You've had your balloon popped and now it's painfully clear that you're not superhuman. This could be a variety of different things. It could be an injury. That's a pretty common one. Or it could be that you haven't made any progress in two years. That's a REALLY common one. You've continued training your butt off and giving it everything you have, but your results haven't improved. Whatever the actual cause is, something has happened to burst your bubble when you're in stage three. You've learned that you actually didn't know everything like you thought in stage two, and you're not at the highest level of knowledge and experience in the sport. To put it very simply, you've been humbled. If we're comparing this to real-life experience, this might be like a time when you're now an adult and you've been burned by something. Maybe it was a divorce, an arrest for DUI, or maybe you got fired from a job. You've been knocked for a loop, and you have to ask yourself, "Where do I go from here?"

Coaches and athletes, please pay close attention to what I'm going to say next.

Stage three is the end of the road for many lifters. The defeat they experienced, whatever it was, proved to be too much for them and they decided to hang it up. They let it beat them. If you've made it to stage three in your career either as a lifter or a coach, I can guarantee that you've at least thought about quitting. It crosses your mind, and you can't believe that it might actually be coming to an end. I think anybody who has been in this sport for an extended period of time has had moments when they thought about walking away. Brothers and sisters, this is when you really start to learn about being a weightlifter. All those little motivational slogans you've seen on gym wall posters over the years, the ones that say things like "It's not how many times you fall, but how many times you get up," you know the ones I'm talking about? Stage three is when those words become reality. You've fallen, and you have to find a way to get up. Nobody can help you, either. The only thing you have to rely on is the strength of your own character. Olympic champion Yuri Zacharevich once said, "There is simply a time in your life when you must clench your teeth and hang on." All of you experienced lifters and coaches who are reading this, do you know what I mean? I know you do. All of you newbies and greenhorns, do you know what I mean? Probably not, but you will someday.

Stage Four: Rebirth

This is the stage you hit when you've survived stage three. You took your lumps, got back to work, and found a way to become successful again. This is where you're finally mature. You've come back from your defeat and now you know that you don't know everything, and you never did in the first place. In fact, you know now that you'll never know everything because the world of weightlifting is a big complex place, and you've also learned that some of the old fogies who you dismissed in stage two probably knew more about weightlifting than you thought they did because they've been through stage three, maybe even more than once. Mark Twain described this time with his famous quote, "When I was a boy of fourteen, my father was so ignorant I could barely stand to have the old man around. But when I got to be twenty-one, I was astonished at how much the old man had learned in seven years."

You might not lift the biggest weights of your life when you're in stage four. You probably hit those when you were in stage two. But there's a difference between lifting the biggest lifts of your life and doing the best lifting of your life. I hit the biggest weights of my life when I was twenty-six, but I think I did some of the best lifting of my career ten years later as a master. My lifts as a master were much lighter than my lifetime bests, but being able to still snatch over 300 pounds and qualify for the Senior Nationals when I was thirty-six years old was, in my mind, some of the finest lifting I've done in my career. Believe me, I had to survive a lot of stage threes along the way. But those stage three moments are the things that have made this whole journey so much more rewarding. If you're a coach, you'll probably never have a greater experience than when you help an athlete make it through stage three, because this is where you learn that this whole road we're traveling is about much more than just lifting weights.

I guess stage four is when you're not a kid anymore. You've been around the block a few times, so to speak. You've had your share of defeats. Nothing is clearer to you at this stage than the knowledge that you're human, just like everybody else. That's a great thing to know in life. What is equally clear to you is the understanding that you should really enjoy and treasure the bright moments of your weightlifting life, because it won't always be sunshine, lemonade and baskets full of puppies. Sometimes, it will be outhouses and spoiled milk. Still, the persistent ones who have fought through stage three and made it to stage four are the ones who reap the biggest rewards. Lemonade tastes a lot sweeter when you've been dying of thirst for a long time.

OUT WITH THE NEW, IN WITH THE OLD

Yesterday, I was walking through a Dick's Sporting Goods store, looking for their prices on iron plates (they're pretty good, incidentally). As I was making my way to the corner of the store where they keep the weight training equipment, I happened to pass through the kids clothing section. I stopped for a couple of minutes as I strolled past the racks of t-shirts, shorts, sweaters, etc. because I noticed something that made me think. The store had several racks of t-shirts with all kinds of little tough-sounding motivational phrases on them. You've all seen the shirts I'm talking about somewhere before, nothing new. But the thing that caught my eye was the actual slogans and words that were on the shirts. I guess we've moved way past the days of shirts that say, "No Pain No Gain" and other overused mottos like that. The shirts I saw yesterday said things like "I feel YOUR pain!" "Dare to take ME on?" and "If you see ME, get used to second place!" As I said, these were all in the kids section of the store, so the shirts were probably meant for ages 9-12, something like that.

After I left the store and started driving to the gym, I found myself thinking a lot about what I saw. All of the words on those shirts were designed to sound cocky, arrogant, self-absorbed, and disrespectful towards other competitors. The store had several racks of them, so it's obvious that these are big sellers. That means that we're living in a culture where parents are putting their kids into sports programs and then buying them clothes that are specially constructed to demonstrate self-worship and insulting attitudes towards opponents. The more I thought about this, the more connection I began to see with much of the adult behavior we see in the sports world today. The NBA is a pretty good place to explain this connection because it's one of the biggest sports venues in the world. Here we find situations where the sport's top stars announce their decisions to switch teams by getting on television and saying things like, "I've decided to take my talents to South Beach." And then when these stars get to South Beach, they hold outrageous spectacles at Miami's American Airlines Arena where they get onstage with two of their teammates (ignoring the rest of their team), and declare themselves "arguably the best trio ever to play the game of basketball." It doesn't stop there, because they have to continue to run their mouths by predicting that they will win "not two, not three, not four" NBA championships. They label themselves as the newest sports dynasty before they've ever played a game together. Yes, I'm talking about LeBron James and the Miami Heat.

So, the process seems clear. Little kids are enrolled in youth basketball, football, soccer, etc. by their parents. Then, their parents buy them the shirts I saw at Dick's so they can try to intimidate the competition. From there, the kids go through their sports careers and the most talented ones make it to the professional level, where they are given the highest possible pedestal to hold glorious celebrations of ME. Their self-absorption and disdain towards others is not only appreciated, but encouraged. Yeah, this sounds about right. Make no mistake about it, professional sports have become a public display stage for the absolute highest levels of selfishness and poor sportsmanship. And since you're all wondering, let me tell you where I'm going with this.

Many of you are coaches, parents, gym owners, etc. In other words, you're in positions where there are people under your instruction. You are an authority figure on some level. This means that you are responsible for teaching and administrating the people you work with. What I want to do with this month's article is examine what kind of job you're doing in these functions. I'm not talking about how you're teaching technique or programming to your athletes or kids, I'm talking about how you're teaching attitude. Let me make it clear right from the beginning that I'm going to be pushing my own personal opinion pretty hard with this one, because this is one area where I'm positive that I'm right. When it comes to training, exercise selection, snatch technique, etc., I've always tried to make it clear that I'm not the only one with the right answers. In this area, however, I think there's a pretty strong distinction between what's right and what's wrong. I'll try to explain my ideas as clearly as possible, and you should be able to find something in here that will make your gym, your home, and your life better.

Old School vs. New School

Everything about our culture has changed over the last hundred years. When people started competing in organized sports around the late 1800s and early 1900s, the personalities of the athletes were reflective of the general attitudes of society. People, for the most part, were much less boisterous and demonstrative than they are now. If you've ever had a chance to watch some of the earliest football, basketball, or weightlifting that was captured on film, you've probably noticed how the athletes acted during competition. There wasn't much celebration or emotion involved. Sure, you would occasionally see athletes jump in the air or raise their hands to the crowd after a successful performance, but it was nothing like the environment today where the sport of football has actually had to invent rules to restrain the celebrations of athletes after they score touchdowns.

This is what we're going to call "old school attitude." An old school attitude was what you saw when athletes just shut their mouths and did their jobs. If they won, they would probably show a little excitement and appreciation to the spectators, but there was definitely a sense of restraint and modesty. If they lost, they shook the hands of their competitors and blamed only themselves for their failure. There was no end zone dancing, choreographed celebration that lasted two minutes, or whining about bad referees after a loss. These types of behaviors were simply not part of the picture because they were considered undignified and self-indulgent.

Smack-talking was often part of the picture with old school athletes, but it was done between the competitors and away from the public. There's no doubt that many great athletes from the days of yore, like Babe Ruth, Jack Johnson, and Norb Schemansky, engaged in some trash talk with their competitors. However, it was different then than it is now. Even if modern technology would have been present beck in 1948, I seriously doubt if you would have ever seen Tommy Kono getting on television and bragging that he was going to win "not two, not three, not four" Olympic medals. The attitude was simply different in those days. You just didn't do stuff like that.

However, fast-forward to 2011 and we've got the disgraceful type of narcissistic circus we see in so many modern sports. We'll call it the "new school attitude," where athletes brag as loudly as possible to as many people as they can, ridicule and insult their competitors, value themselves more than their teams, and refuse to take personal responsibility when they fail. If you watch ESPN long enough, you'll get a pretty good idea of what I'm talking about. Now, let me make it clear that not every athlete in the modern era has been contaminated by the new school attitude. I was just watching a Grand Slam tennis tournament last month where Rafael Nadal beat Roger Federer for the championship. The behavior of both these men was a pretty classy demonstration of old school behavior, as Nadal complimented Federer after the match by saying, "I respect Roger because he acts the same whether he wins or loses." These guys are clear examples of positive athletic behavior, and they're not the only ones in contemporary sports that act right. But the fact still remains that you can't watch sports for very long these days without seeing something that just makes you want to vomit because of how immature and negative it is.

When did everything change? When did we go from old school to new school? It's not something that happed instantaneously or because of one person, but I do personally believe that Muhammad Ali had a lot to do with changing the sports culture in this country. Ali was one of the greatest athletes in history, and his accomplishments in boxing were equaled only by his incredible personality. Ali's trash talking, disrespect towards his opponents, and self-promotion were done at a level that had never been seen in sports before. His image was so larger-than-life that he heavily influenced generations of young athletes that have grown up in his wake. Kids have actually moved through their athletic careers wanting to embody the same showmanship and bravado that Ali had. He is the point of origin for much of the new school attitude. Please understand, though, that I'm not committing the sacrilege of dumping on Muhammad Ali here. As an athlete, I hold Ali on a pedestal as one of the supreme competitors I've ever seen. I never liked his behavior and I still don't, but I would never deny his greatness as an athlete.

Therefore, we have a stark contrast between two very different methods. Based on how I've described all of this, you can probably guess where I stand in the evaluation of old school vs. new school. I am very much an old school personality, I require my athletes to be the same way, and I reject new school attitude as being childish, irresponsible, and shameful. Got it? Hopefully I made that clear enough. But then that leaves us with you. What kind of personality are you, and what are you doing to make sure your athletes, children, etc. are developing in the right direction? Let's take a look at this, and I'll give you a few handy dandy tips to make sure you're not contributing to the ramming of modern sports into the toilet.

The basic blueprint for not becoming a jerkoff

How do you represent yourself in the strength world? Because one thing you better believe is that when you're a coach, your personality will filter down into your athletes. Even if you're not a coach, your personality still will filter down to the other lifters in your gym, your children, friends who admire you, etc. There's a sense of accountability that has to be there. If you're in any position of authority or responsibility, the people around you will often act the way you act.

I've used the word "selfishness" quite a few times in this article, and obviously there's been a negative connotation with it. However, I should mention that being selfish is very important to an elite athlete. If you're in a position where you're competing at the top of your sport, you have to have a certain element of self-centeredness to be successful. High-level athletes have to see their training and their performance as the most important things in the universe. These aren't always the most endearing people to be around because they basically expect the whole world to stop and revolve around their workouts. For better or worse, this just comes with the territory. Championship athletes usually aren't very giving personalities. Hopefully, that all changes after retirement or once age sets in and real life gets started. Most elite athletes go through a lot of attitude changes when they make the transition to civilian life, and that's a good thing.

The negative aspect of selfishness that I'm describing here is the point where selfishness makes the transition to blatant punk behavior. It's fine to be totally focused on your athletic priorities, but we need to make sure that we don't cross over into the bragging, impertinence, and whining. Hell, I'll make this easy for you. Here are four simple things you can do that will keep you from looking like a turd:

Show a lot of interest, enthusiasm, and support for others. Simplest thing in the world, right? Just start caring and getting excited about the people around you. You will absolutely never go wrong if you cheer for others during their workouts, congratulate them after they're successful, and throw them a little encouragement when they're down. This is 100% guaranteed stuff and it takes very little energy.

Don't talk about your accomplishments unless somebody asks you about them. The quickest way to make a bad first impression is to start throwing your resume in somebody's face without any reason. If you're a stud, people will either already know it when they meet you or they'll figure it out pretty quickly. You don't need to wave your gold medals around your head. It looks insecure and arrogant.

Don't coach people in the gym unless they ask for it. Let's say you're in a gym training and you see somebody who's clearly doing something wrong. If the person has a coach who is working with them, you need to just stay out of it. It's none of your business, so don't turn into to Butty McButtinstein. Now, if the person doesn't have a coach and they're doing something wrong, just ask them "Do you mind if I give you a suggestion?" You'll know pretty fast if they want to listen to you or not, and then you can proceed accordingly. If it's obvious that they want you to keep your comments to yourself, then do it. You asked politely, so you're in the clear.

Don't get on the internet and talk @%!* Ooohhh, I think I'm probably ruffling some feathers with this one. Look, the internet is the greatest medium in the history of civilization for people who want to unleash their anger and disgust over how stupid everybody else in the world is. But even if you're right and your opponent is wrong, you'll both still come away from the argument looking stupid. Just don't do it baby.

Quick Confession: Just so nobody calls me a hypocrite or thinks I'm sitting on my high horse, I'll openly admit that I've violated every one of these suggestions at some point in my life. Nobody's perfect.

In Conclusion…

A lot of the mistakes that come with new school attitude are connected with youth. It's pretty easy to act like a dork when you're young. We've all done it. It's part of growing up. And you coaches need to remember this because most kids literally don't know how they're supposed to act. We sometimes make the mistake of telling ourselves, "Dammit, they should know better than that!" Well, maybe they DON'T know better than that. Maybe nobody has ever told them the difference between acting right and acting wrong. Remember, some of these kids you work with have been practically raised by wolves. They need some guidance.

And as always, I know there's the possibility that some of you might think everything I've just said is all wrong. If you just got back from Dick's Sporting Goods and you're excited to give little ten year-old Tyler a shirt you just bought him that says, "I'm number one and everybody can lick my butthole" so he can wear it to youth wrestling practice tomorrow, then I guess we probably have a difference in opinion. But here's some food for thought. What if Tyler shows up to wrestling practice with his cocky new shirt, and then he gets pinned in sixteen seconds by some tough little Mormon kid? At that point, we can safely say that Tyler is NOT number one, and that shirt is gonna look pretty stupid. Don't humiliate your kids.

Look, I'm not telling you to be boring. I'm not telling you that you have to be an emotionless robot as an athlete, and I'm certainly not telling you that you can't have a colorful personality. We don't have to stay stuck in the Stone Age; we couldn't even if we wanted to. Times change, and you have to be able to keep up with the changes. But not all changes are good. The shift we've seen towards total self-absorption and egotism is not good. Whining is not good. Insulting your competitors is not good. So do society a favor and take a stand against those things. Make your athletes take a stand against them too, and maybe we'll all have a better experience in our sports lives. Let's give it a try.

AND DOGGONE IT, PEOPLE LIKE ME!

When I was in college, I took a class called Human Relations Development. The course was required for my education major, and this was the touchy-feely class to end all touchy-feely classes. The professor was a very kind little old man who spoke in a gentle tone and usually patted you on the shoulder at least a few times when you were talking with him. The whole focus of the class was to make future teachers more skilled at communicating with people, listening attentively to their problems, gaining their trust, finding effective ways to assist them with their troubles, etc. You get the idea. It was a class about sensitivity.

As a twenty-two year old weightlifting male with a football background and a testosterone level that seemed to grow by the hour, I was way out of my element here. Most of the other students were women, and men with personalities that closely resembled women. One of the first lessons we completed in the class was an exercise that determined what kind of problem-solvers we were. If I described the whole exercise to you, your boredom would rapidly approach the jumping-out-of-a-window-to-end-it-all level. But the end result of the exercise told me that I was rated as a lousy, unproductive, insensitive problem-solver. I couldn't understand why my rating was so low, either. To my way of thinking, there was a simple way of handling people when they had problems. My basic idea was, "Tell me what the hell is wrong, then I'll tell you how to fix it, then you take your head out of your butthole and do what I say." I thought this sounded like a pretty solid approach.

Anyway, the class dragged on and I managed to get an A despite the fact that I didn't really change much. I learned how to fake the "nice and caring" thing pretty well, but I was still a calloused meathead when it was all over. Now, fast-forward sixteen years, I'm thirty-eight years old and I think my professor would be proud of me. A couple of marriages and fifteen years of coaching have forced me to actually learn how to listen to people and care about their feelings. I'm like the freakin' Dr. Phil of weightlifting. Because of my transformation, I'm going to write this month's article about an idea that was recently suggested to me by a very sharp lady. She thought it would be interesting to write about the topic of coachability from the perspective of the athlete. In other words, we're talking about "what an athlete should look for in a coach and how to handle different issues that arise" between coaches and athletes (I'm actually quoting her e-mail to me). *What should an athlete want from a coach?* That's the question we're going to answer. And to prove even further what a wonderful human being I am, I'm even going to address the exact categories she suggested. We'll look at specific traits that are essential in coaching and also a few hazards that athletes should be wary of. If this isn't caring and considerate, then I don't know what the hell is. Please keep reading, and feel free to bask in the warmth of my empathy.

Category 1

Eye for technique/ability to explain things clearly Needless to say, this quality is absolutely, positively necessary for anyone who wants to coach the Olympic Lifts. The coach has to have a complete understanding of how a snatch or clean and jerk should look and feel. This is usually developed through years of experience in the sport. Most of the best coaches are people with a large range of experience in both lifting and coaching. It takes years to learn exactly how a snatch is supposed to feel and how to make your body execute the correct movements to make it happen. After that, it also takes years to learn exactly what a snatch is supposed to look like and how to make someone else's body execute the correct movements to make it happen. When I was young and getting started in my weightlifting career, I wanted to be coached by someone who had actually been a weightlifter. It was important to me that my coach had walked the walk as an athlete. My faith in the coach would be stronger if I knew he had trained and competed at a high level. This may or may not be important to other athletes. There are certainly some very successful coaches who were not high-level athletes themselves. And clearly, there are also many high-level athletes who couldn't coach their way out of a wet paper bag with their hands on fire. Basically, the athlete's individual perspective on their coach is what matters in this area.

Regardless of competitive experience on the part of the coach, the one area that is indispensable is the coach's ability to TEACH. The best coaches are great teachers. A coach can be a former world record holder and it won't make a lick of difference if he/she doesn't have the ability to clearly explain to the athletes what they're supposed to be doing. This is where I believe that most great coaches are very organized in their thinking. When dealing with a lifter who has previously learned the lifts and needs coaching to get better, the coach looks at the athlete and immediately identifies which areas need to be corrected and which ones are already solid. One of the phrases I use with athletes is, "Okay, you're already doing a lot of things right. Now here's one area I think we need to fix." (Hint: Always start with a positive comment and always say "we" when you're working with an athlete. Athletes like to believe that the two of you are in it together.) Good coaches fix one problem at a time. If you give an athlete three or four technical suggestions at the same time, they'll probably get confused. And please don't start off with some kind of negative comment like, "Jeez, you're a total mess." It doesn't accomplish anything productive and some people are sensitive.

They'll immediately think they're a piece of crap when you say things like that. Then you've lost them.

Category 2

Being open to suggestions from other areas My perspective on this area might surprise you and many of you definitely might disagree with it. In my experience, most of the best coaches are control freaks who are fairly inflexible in their methods. They're usually not very open to suggestions from other areas. Now, the general mental flow of our society tells us that people have to work together to be successful. Corporate methodology in the workplace is usually based on idea sharing, think tank principles, and bosses who are open to input from employees. That's the modern way. Dictatorships aren't popular nowadays.

However, I think coaching is an area where this rule has to get broken. Great coaches usually have a dictator mentality. When coaches spend years building a successful methodology and then use this methodology to consistently produce outstanding results, they usually don't welcome alternate ideas from outside sources. I coach track and field for a living and one of the things I say to my athletes every year at our first-day meeting is, "Make sure you understand something. This is a my-way-or-the-highway program. I'm the coach and you're the athletes, and you're going to do what I tell you to do. This might sound like a dictatorship, and that's what it is. But you also need to understand that you'll benefit from this, because the way I coach you is going to make you better. If you do what I tell you to do, you're going to be successful." Over the course of the season, I blend this approach with a lot of humor. I also let the athletes know in every possible way that I care about them, I respect them, and I'm committed to their success not only in track and field, but in life. This has worked for me. I'm a control freak, and I make them believe that's a good thing.

But as with anything else, there are special considerations to keep in mind when discussing dictator-type coaching. First of all, most of the best international weightlifting coaches in history have come from communist societies where the people are already adjusted to the idea of submitting to government control. This is America, where you're going to encounter some very willful personalities. That skews things just a bit. Also, working with adults is different from working with young people. You can't treat an adult like a sixteen-year-old kid and expect them to stick around for long. If you push the totalitarian attitude too hard, you'll turn people off. My general advice to athletes is that the coach is the boss, and you have to be willing to obey the coach if you want to have a successful relationship. That doesn't mean that you have to tremble in fear and prostrate yourself when the coach walks in the gym, but it does mean that you have to be a disciplined pupil. If you were coached by a legend like John Wooden, Vince Lombardi, or Ivan Abadjiev, you would have no question about who was running the show when you came to practice every day. This is a good thing.

Category 3

Work ethic This one is easy. As a coach, how can you ask an athlete to work hard if you're not willing to show up every day and work hard yourself? If you're lazy, you're going to lose athletes quickly and you have nobody to blame but yourself. Simple enough? Good, then let's move on.

Category 4

Personality Aahhh, the glue that holds it all together. How can I say this clearly? Let's put it this way: when you enter into a coach-athlete relationship with somebody, you're making a commitment to spend a large portion of your life with that person. You're going to be around each other all the time. *There's no way this can work if the athlete doesn't like the coach.* In fact, I would even go so far as to say that there will never be maximum results unless the athlete LOVES the coach. When I say "love," I'm obviously not talking about romantic feelings and passionate experience (this is unprofessional and it's usually one great big recipe for disaster, by the way). I'm talking about the type of love family members share with each other. I've been lucky in my sports life to have a couple of coaches who I felt this way about, and I've been incredibly lucky to coach a lot of athletes in the same way. When you get one of those rare situations where the coach and the athlete truly believe in each other, and both of them would sweat blood for the other one, then you've got something special. If you throw some athletic talent and coaching expertise into this mix, then you're going to be looking at some championships.

Coaches have to be driven to make their athletes better, but the best coaches are the ones who impact their athletes' lives in a much deeper way. Athletes want to know their coaches care about them. If the coach doesn't care, you can bet your bottom dollar that the athletes will figure it out rapidly. Now, can coaches and athletes have success if they don't share this type of deep bond? Sure they can. If a coach is talented and the athlete is committed, then the results will be positive even if it's just a business-type relationship.

But if the athlete simply doesn't like the coach, then it's a dead duck. The relationship might work for a while if the athlete is a particularly tolerant person, but it will eventually sour. Also, make sure you remember that there's a difference between liking/loving somebody and being pissed off at them. You can love somebody and still get angry with them from time to time. If you want to truly learn this, get married. Coaches and athletes will have the same types of experiences. It's not all going to be baskets full of puppies and pineapple ice cream, believe me. If you're in a weightlifting coach-athlete relationship with somebody, you're going to have moments when you want to attack them with an ice pick. But once the anger subsides and everybody cools off, how do you really feel about your coach? If you still have loyalty and respect for your coach/athlete despite the rough moments and you still believe that you're with the right person, then you've got a good thing going. If you take an honest look at the big picture and you decide that you simply don't like the person, then it's time to move on. If there are no other coaches in your area to train with, then it gets really tricky. You'll need to get creative at that point.

When we come full circle, it's clear that a good coach has to have a special combination of qualities. It's not an easy gig, and it takes a lot of trial and error to perfect it. If you're an athlete and you want to say something to your coach, go ahead and say it. Make sure you pick the right time, obviously. Any coach worth a plug nickel will do exactly what I was taught to do in my Human Relations Development class... LISTEN. Now, you (the athlete) also need to be prepared if the answer isn't exactly what you wanted to hear. If you want a coach, but you also want to be the one running the show, then you need to back up and examine your own personality. The coach isn't the problem at that point. You are.

But my guess is that if you and your coach both have sensible, functional personalities, then the two of you will most likely be able to work together. If you have any tough times, try using an exercise where you both sit down and write a poem about each other. That sounds like a special way to share sensitive feelings of happiness. Just don't start your poem with the line, "There once was a man from Nantucket..."

COACHES AREN'T THAT IMPORTANT... RIGHT?

One of the best pizzas I've ever had in my life was from a little Greek place in Seattle called Santorini's. Tiny hole-in-the-wall restaurant, Greek owned and operated, and I've been saying for years that they put out one of the best pies I've ever chomped on. Anyway, I remember sitting in this joint several years ago, feasting and having beers with a friend of mine. This friend was an elite American lifter from the 80s...World Team member, American record-holder, the whole bit. He and I were in the middle of a conversation about former Olympic gold medalists in weightlifting who had gone into coaching after their athletic careers were over, and how many of them had been successful. It was a fun few minutes of weightlifting trivial pursuit while we tried to recall how many top lifters had gone on to become top coaches. Names like Alexeev, Suleymanoglu, Rigert, Kono, and other superstars come to mind, and we diagnosed how effective their coaching had been based on their country's world championship performance. In the middle of this conversation, I asked my buddy if he thought world champion lifters made good coaches. His answer was, "I don't know. Coaching is overrated anyway."

"Coaching is overrated." I've been thinking about that statement for fifteen years. The point he was making was that athletes either have the natural ability to become champions or they don't, plain and simple. The ones that have world championship ability will probably become world champions regardless of who their coach is because they simply have more talent than anybody in the world. And the ones that don't have world championship ability? You could give them the best coaching in the planet throughout their entire careers, and they'll never make it to the top. That was the general idea of the dinner banter.

I'm a coach, as many of you are. One of the beliefs that I think is common among all coaches is that we control how successful our athletes are. If they win championships, it's because we guided them to those championships. If they fail, it's because we didn't prepare them properly. The statement "coaching is over-rated" punches a few holes in our basic belief system, because it basically says that we're just not as important as we think we are. I think this is damn fine material for an article. And as with most of the subjects we analyze here at *Performance Menu*, it's not a simple black-and-white issue. Like a good pizza, there are many different components involved.

Big Al and his Magic Towel…

Does everybody here know who Al Oerter was? Probably not, which is a shame. Al Oerter was one of the greatest athletes who ever lived, no question about it. An American discus thrower, Al won four Olympic gold medals. That's right, four of them. Even more impressive is the fact that Al set new Olympic records in all four of these performances, and he won a couple of them with torn cartilage in his ribs, neck injuries, etc. Al's greatness is beyond comparison, and one of the freaky things about him is that he was never really coached in his career. He basically taught himself. I heard an interview with him once where he was asked who his coach was throughout his prime years. Al said, "My coach was a towel."

What the heck does that mean? Al went on to explain that he didn't have a coach. All he did was set a towel out in the throwing sector at the distance he wanted to hit with the discus. If he wanted to throw 190 feet, for example, he would just take a white gym towel and lay it on the ground 190 feet from the disc ring. Then, he would just go through his workout and make sure he threw past the towel. No coaching, no input from others, no video, etc. He just put a towel out there and made sure he threw the discus past it. Using this method, he won Olympic gold four times. Seriously guys, I'm not making this up. The guy was from another galaxy.

Now, there are some things that we have to openly acknowledge about this example. Clearly, Al Oerter had a level of natural talent that was beyond human comprehension. The "towel method" worked for him because he simply didn't need much help from anybody. He was born with an unnatural sense of knowing how to make his body move in the most effective pattern, and he also happened to have the strength, power, balance, and coordination to perfect that pattern. These things are obvious. Equally obvious is the fact that athletes like Al Oerter are extraordinarily rare. People just aren't born with tools like this on a regular basis.

However, Al isn't the only example in history. Olympic weightlifting legend Vasily Alexeev was very similar. Alexeev won two Olympic gold medals and broke eighty world records during his ten-year reign of invincibility in the 70s. Like Al, Vasily trained alone and formed his own methodology. He was able to dominate the world for a very long time without any coaching, just by doing his own thing. In addition to these two men, there have been a few other cases throughout sports history where athletes reach world record greatness without being coached. However, do these examples prove to us that coaching is overrated or, perhaps, unnecessary? Well… here's another angle we have to look at.

Ivan Abadjiev

Okay, most of you probably didn't know who Al Oerter was. How about Ivan Abadjiev, do any of you know who he is? Anyone? Anyone? Dang it, I hope you're not zero for two. If you are, let me bring you up to speed. Ivan Abadjiev was the head national coach of the Bulgarian weightlifting team during the 70s, 80s, and early 90s. Bulgaria, in case you don't know, is a relatively small European country with very little weightlifting success prior to the early 70s when Abadjiev was hired. This man built Bulgaria into one of the most feared powerhouses in the history of the sport. The 80s were an insane rampage of world champions and world records from this tiny nation, as they toppled the massive Soviet Union to become the best weightlifting team on the planet. Abadjiev is widely considered the greatest coach in the history of the sport, and there is no question that he was an iron-fisted control freak who ran his program with a dictator mentality. Abadjiev's belief was that his program would produce world champions, plain and simple. He understood that most athletes would not be able to handle the inhuman workload of his training program. But the ones that could handle it would become the best in the world. And it worked.

This is an interesting contrast to the examples of Oerter and Alexeev. With those two men, you had a situation where coaching was irrelevant. They had their success with nobody telling them what to do. With Abadjiev and the Bulgarians, however, the level of success was almost entirely attributed to the coach. Through his vision and his direction, the national program was developed into a weightlifting machine. Year after year, the Bulgarians simply pumped new bodies into the machine the way meat is pumped into a sausage grinder. With Abadjiev cranking the handle, the Bulgarian program spit out world champions as reliably as the grinder churned out sausages.

We have examples where championships are won without any coaching at all. And then we have other examples where coaching is almost the sole reason for the championships. So, getting back to our original question, is coaching overrated?

It's All About Levels…

The answer to this question has to be a little long-winded, so let's break it down in a way that makes it easy to understand. Let's take a look at different levels of athletes:

Al and Alexeev Level With these athletes, coaching isn't even necessary. They have so many God-given gifts that they can simply operate on their own and they will still rise to the top of their sport. Okay, we understand. And we also understand that athletes at this level are one-in-a-trillion. They're the Haley's Comets of sports.

Not quite Al and Alexeev but still way ahead of everybody else Level Here, we're looking at athletes who are extremely talented, but they still need coaching and direction. These are freaky studs, but they don't quite have the athletic genius to be able to operate on their own. The interesting thing about these athletes is that they will usually be successful no matter who their coach is. As long as they're being coached by somebody who knows the basics of training and knows how to manage personalities, these athletes will win championships. Their success doesn't come from their coach, not really. Their success comes from their natural gifts, and their coach is more of a "talent manager" than anything else. If you happen to work with athletes like this in your coaching career, the best advice I can give you is "don't over-coach them." These athletes will need much less input and instruction than most other athletes. With these cats, the coach basically just needs to make sure they train consistently and show up for the competition on time. These are the ones that make life easy.

The Massive Majority Level Now we're talking about the area that almost all of your athletes will fall into. This is the level where the athlete has solid athletic talent and good work ethic, but they will not rise to the top without very well-planned training and preparation. These athletes don't have the same physical gifts as the athletes in the two higher levels that we just examined. And to be totally realistic about it, these athletes should not be able to beat the athletes in the two higher levels. However, this is where life can get interesting. Because if you have Massive Majority Level athletes who have astonishing work ethic and amazing commitment, and they're competing against Al and Alexeev Level athletes who have unparalleled physical gifts but also happen to be lazy and stupid, then you might just have a shot. Massive Majority athletes are not supposed to beat Al and Alexeev athletes, make no mistake about it. Donkeys don't usually outrun thoroughbred race horses in the Kentucky Derby. But if the coach, the program, and the mental qualities of the Massive Majority athletes are exceptional enough, then there could be exceptional results.

Genetic Cesspool Level Groan… These are the athletes who, God bless them, just don't have it. They can barely stand up straight and cough at the same time. You could coach these poor critters until judgment day and they'll never win championships. You'll know these athletes when you see them. And you want to know the hardest part of it all? These athletes often have the highest work-ethic, commitment, and love for what they're doing. They suck and they know it, but they freaking love the sport and they'll bust their butts harder than anybody. Some coaches turn these athletes away, and I say shame on them for doing that. Because one thing I can tell you for sure is that these athletes can very easily become your best volunteers, most loyal supporters, and most faithful contributors. I always tell people that if they work hard, contribute something to the program, and don't cause trouble, then they're welcome members of the team. You should do the same.

Are we ever gonna get an answer?

"Coaching is overrated." True or false? We can say that this statement has some truth to it. At the end of the day, an athlete's talent level will be the deciding factor in his/her career. Average is not supposed to beat exceptional. Superior shouldn't lose to normal. These things are true, and coaching doesn't have much to do with it. I've seen some really phenomenal athletes who are coached by borderline incompetents. The athletes still win championships because they're just better than everybody else. Nothing complicated about it.

However, the best coaches are the ones who build great programs. A great program is one that produces high-level results year after year, even if there aren't any Al Oerters or Vasily Alexeevs running around. Abadjiev built Bulgaria into this type of program. Now, it's obvious that there were a lot of exceptional athletes in the Bulgarian program throughout the 70s and 80s. You can't be a world champion without being an exceptional athlete. But the point is that the Bulgarians achieved the highest levels of success for many years, and that success was driven by the coach who set the whole operation up.

One thing I would say about great coaches is that they can design effective training programs, but even more important than the program is the environment they create. Great coaches create great training environments. The "environment" is the atmosphere of discipline, enthusiasm, intensity, and respect for the team that you see when you walk in a gym. This is, in my opinion, the most important element of coaching. Athletes have to be able to actually feel a sense of responsibility and high expectation when the coach is present. They have to feel like everything is under control when the coach is there, because that is the feeling that will propel them forward to greater results. If a coach is panicky, disagreeable, or negative, then the athletes will develop those same qualities. Pretty soon, you've just got a gym full of losers.

Is coaching overrated? Well, I guess we can admit that nobody every turned horse manure into pancakes just by pouring syrup on it. None of the JV discus throwers on the track team I coach will probably ever break Al Oerter's record of four Olympic gold medals. But if I do my job as a coach, I might be able to get that JV thrower into the finals of the state championship in three years. At that point, we've seen exceptional results from an average kid. That, my friends, is where coaching is most definitely NOT overrated. We took something normal and we turned it into something special, just like a great pizza maker does. Anybody can spin dough and then toss some toppings on it. But think about the best pizza you've ever had in your life. Go ahead, think about it right now. That pizza was perfect because somebody took a bunch of ordinary ingredients and made something amazing from them. Not just any hick from the street could make that pizza taste as great as it did. It was great because it was made by a master. That's coaching, and it makes all the difference in the world.

CONCLUSION

When I was a young kid, my father gave me a bible. Inside the cover, he wrote me a short note. Although I haven't seen this bible in at least fifteen years, I remember the note. It said:

> *Son, look for two things in this book:*
> Truth
> Yourself
> *You will find both.*

And right now, some of you are shaking your heads and saying, "Holy crap, Matt's gonna compare this book to the bible." No, no… that's not where I'm going with this.

But I definitely will compare the journey of a strength athlete to a spiritual quest. I figured out a long time ago that my obsession with lifting weights wasn't just about getting big and strong. For me, it was always about something much more than that. I think the reason weightlifting meant so much to me in the early days is that it gave me a chance to beat away the self-doubt and insecurity I had as a teenager. Succeeding as a lifter was a way for me to believe in myself. I firmly believe that most people want to be a part of something special. The sport of weightlifting and the community of the iron world served that purpose for me, and it still does. Lifting weights is about much more than strengthening your body. It's about strengthening your spirit and your personality.

Now, I've been very fortunate in my life to have a loving family that I'm very close to, an awesome wife, and a job that gives me a lot of happiness on a daily basis. Those are the great things of my life. My beliefs in religion, faith, and spirituality have taken a lot of twists and turns over the years. I've been hot and I've been cold in that department. But one area where I've never grown cold is weightlifting. Even when things have been bad… times of stagnation, injuries, losing some strength to Father Time… I've still never had a moment when I didn't love it. I love training and I love helping other people learn the sport and improve. I also love the people who have helped me throughout my weightlifting career, and there have been a lot of them. Being a member of the Calpian Weightlifting Club and training for John Thrush have been some of the great privileges of my life. All of the training partners and friends I've known, the undying support of my parents, the other contributors to the sport that have helped me either directly or indirectly, the great people from the past who have built the foundations of the lifting world. Sometimes I can't believe how lucky I am.

I'm glad you decided to read this. Now that you've finished it, I recommend going deeper into your lifting life. Read as much as you can, learn as much as you can, and help others as much as you can. I'll continue writing for The Performance Menu until it shuts down, Greg and Aimee fire me, or I run out of things to say. I hope you keep reading, because we all still have a long way to go on the iron road. And we're all in it together.